FALLING IN LOVE
WITH THE PROCESS

Cultivating Resilience in Health Crises

A Stroke Survivor's Story

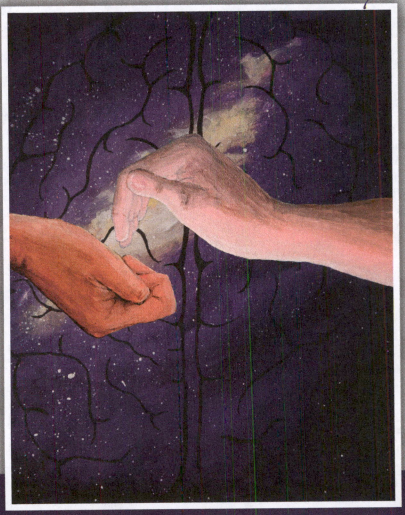

Sarah Parsloe, Ph.D. | Patricia Geist-Martin, Ph.D.

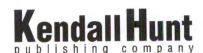

Kendall Hunt
publishing company

Cover designer: Brianne Fortier

DESCRIPTION OF FRONT COVER ARTIST BRIANNE FORTIER AND HER ART
Brianne Fortier's artwork has been an ever-evolving creative process. Having grown up in Iowa, her early artworks are very much inspired by the beautiful scenery that surrounded her while living on her family's farm. After graduating with a BA in Biology, Brianne moved to San Diego, earning her MA in Communication. When Patricia and Sarah approached her to paint a piece for their cover, she was thrilled that she could combine her love for science with her art. Brianne listened to Sarah and Patricia describe what happens to the brain and, specifically, to neural connections when a stroke survivor re-learns the process of moving their fingers. It became clear to her that she needed to make the hands a focal point for this piece. The galaxy as the background was what Brianne envisioned to represent the neurons making connections and "lighting up" as the stroke survivor begins to recover.

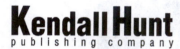

Kendall Hunt
publishing company

www.kendallhunt.com
Send all inquiries to:
4050 Westmark Drive
Dubuque, IA 52004-1840

Copyright © 2020 by Kendall Hunt Publishing Company

ISBN 978-1-5249-8989-7

Published in the United States of America.

CONTENTS

PROLOGUE v

PART 1: PICKING UP THE PIECES; CONNECTING THE DOTS 1

CHAPTER 1. "Something Is Wrong": The Stroke That Changed Everything 3

CHAPTER 2. "Do It to the Best of Your Ability": Cultivating Resilience 11

CHAPTER 3. "I Just Knew I Would Get Better": Waking Up to the Realities of a Stroke 23

CHAPTER 4. "Always Searching for Something": Love, Loss, and the Will to Live 33

CHAPTER 5. "I Wanted to Go Home and Hide": The Emotional Journey of Stroke Recovery 47

CHAPTER 6. "I Was Always One Step Ahead": Memories from "Our Man on Maui" 57

PART 2: PERSISTING THROUGH RECOVERY 75

CHAPTER 7. "If Kirk Douglas Can Do It, So Can I": Persisting in Stroke Recovery 77

CHAPTER 8. "I Just Fell in Love with It": The Birth of a Sport, a Change of Career 89

CHAPTER 9. "Anybody He's Helped Is His Friend Forever":
Recovery through Supportive Friendships 101

CHAPTER 10. "What's My Next Adventure?": From Sailor to Salesman 111

CHAPTER 11. "I'm Always Full of Coincidences": Larger-than-Life Tales of Success 121

PART 3: COMMUNICATING AS AN ADVOCATE 135

CHAPTER 12. "You Sincerely Care about What Happens to Other People":
From Salesman to Advocate 137

CHAPTER 13. Becoming an "Independent Contractor": Advocating Beyond the Hospital 155

CHAPTER 14. "I Set Myself Up for Being Disappointed": The Emotional Challenges of Advocacy 165

CHAPTER 15. "We Shine a Big Light" on Advocates: Expressing Gratitude 183

EPILOGUE 203

PROLOGUE

"WHY ME?" These were the first words that Bill Torres spoke after waking up from his stroke. Like many survivors, Bill lived his first days and weeks after stroke in a dark, heavy cloud of depression. Depression creates feelings of hopelessness, guilt, helplessness, and decreased energy—all symptoms that stand in the way of a survivor's efforts to regain mobility and speech. Yet, rather than dwelling on asking "WHY ME?" Bill's second words were, "WHAT NOW?" He set his mind to getting better, little by little, every day. As researcher and author, Peter Levine (2013) suggests, stroke survivors must "fall in love with the process … [and] see the process of recovery as an opportunity for growth" (p. xiv).

MEETING BILL: PATRICIA'S STORY

It was a beautifully sunny, warm November day in San Diego. I was working out with weights at Lake Murray with four of my friends and my trainer, Laurie. Our workouts were a funfest of gossip, laughter, and a little exercise. There were not many people at the lake during the work week, so it was a quiet, serene place to get in a workout. Just as we were finishing up our routine and chatting together, a man in blue sweats, a red sweatshirt, and a full head of white-gray hair strolled up to our group.

"How are you ladies doing?" the man asked. He looked to be in his 60s. He smiled at each of us as he spoke, the warm tone of his voice carrying a kind of magnetic charisma.

"Just fine," I responded, returning his smile with a slight hesitation. I was not quite sure what to make of the man's approach, but I was amused with his flirtation. "What are you doing here?"

"I come here every single day to feed the ducks," he replied with a bit of pride in his voice. There was no doubt that he was telling us the truth; we were rapidly being surrounded by the gang of ducks, geese, birds, and squirrels that had followed the man over to our space by the picnic table. Soon, we were shouting to each other over the noise of the birds' loud, demanding quacks, chirps, and honks.

"You come here every single day?" I asked, raising my voice above the clatter.

"Haven't missed more than a few days in the five years since my stroke," the man said, tossing out grain to his crowd of duck fans.

"You had a stroke?" I asked, squinting at the man as if he might be lying. He certainly didn't look like what I imagined when I pictured a stroke survivor.

"Yes, when I was 69. I have worked very hard to recover for the past five years," Bill explained.

"Wow, I would never have guessed that you've had a stroke," I gushed. "And I would never have put you in your 70s! Amazing. You are amazing."

This man seemed fascinating; I wanted to know more about his story. I introduced myself as a communication professor at San Diego State University. "I'm Bill Torres," he told me, pulling a business card out of his wallet. The blue card included his name, the words "stroke survivor," and his contact information alongside a picture of him feeding the ducks.

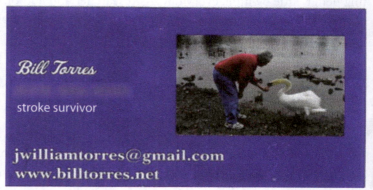

Bill's business card

Immediately, I realized how great it would be to have Bill come and speak to my Health Communication class about his journey from stroke to recovery.

"I'd love to," Bill replied when I asked if he might guest lecture. "But I have one request. Sharp Hospital made this video about my recovery for a program called *Victories of Spirit*. Would you show that video first? Then I can walk in—the real deal—and the students will be surprised to see the kind of recovery I have made."

"Sure, that would be perfect!" I said, getting excited about his visit. I looked at Bill and then back at his card. "Should I call you or e-mail you?"

"Either one is fine. I am retired and, other than my commitment to feed the ducks every day, I am open to when you would need me to come into your class."

By this time, my workout buddies had packed our weights into the car and gathered around us, wanting to learn more about this mystery man. Bill was taken with all the attention—until the birds started landing on his shoulders and pecking at the bag of birdseed he held in one hand. One pigeon even decided to land on his head! It was a sign that it was time to leave, but I promised Bill that I would give him a call soon.

***

That's how I met Bill Torres, over 10 years ago. At least once a year, he gives an hour-long presentation to my Health Communication class. Every year the students say the same thing: "Bill's was the best presentation all semester." He has stiff competition; my lineup of speakers often includes physicians, midwives, hospice staff, and other health-related professionals. Students become even more enamored with Bill when he holds up his SDSU ID, showing that he earned his BA in Education in 1962 and that he paid only US$20.25 in student fees.

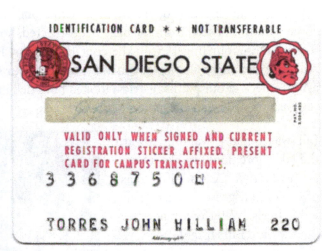

Bill's San Diego State University ID

Over our time together, Bill learned that I had already written four books. He suggested that we might write together about stroke recovery and advocacy. The idea was a good one, but I wasn't quite ready to dive in. I kept delaying the project, but Bill would not let up on his campaign. "You've gotta write this book before I die. C'mon!" he'd say. His tone was humorous, but his words were still quite persuasive. I contemplated the idea. I knew it would be more fun and an easier task if I shared the work with a collaborator. One of my former masters' students, Sarah Parsloe, was just about to complete her PhD dissertation focusing on advocacy, disability, and chronic illness. I proposed the idea of the book to her. Soon, Sarah was boarding a plane heading from her new home in Orlando to San Diego, flying out to meet Bill herself.

MEETING BILL: SARAH'S STORY

Meeting Bill Torres is like meeting a close family member that you haven't seen in a very long time. At least, that's how it felt to me that first time I accompanied Patricia to meet Bill at his new duck-feeding spot in Chollas Lake Park. It was just after 7 a.m. when we pulled into the parking lot. The sky was still the gray-blue color of early morning. It transformed the lake into a silver mirror set amidst brown dirt hiking trails covered in the dried leaves of pale-barked eucalyptus trees. Bill had already arrived. He was standing near the open trunk of a tiny red Fiat, removing large bags of birdseed and roasted peanuts. A few brazen pigeons were already swooping around him, hovering expectantly.

"You must be Sarah," Bill said, joining us as we climbed out of Patricia's Honda. He shook my hand, holding my cold fingers in his warm grasp for an extra beat as he looked into my eyes appraisingly. Bill told me later that he's quite particular about handshakes—he only shakes a person's hand when he feels a connection with them.

"Hey, Patricia!" Bill added, greeting her with a one-armed hug. "Well, the ducks are hungry! Grab some handfuls of seed from the bag," he instructed, holding out the sack in his other hand. We each dug in, filling our fingers with the cool, dry grains. Pigeons descended on us immediately. Their scaly feet and sharp claws grabbed at the fabric of our sweatshirt sleeves as they landed on our forearms to peck at our palms. Patricia looked both delighted and unnerved. She flinched as she heard the rush of birds' wings flapping next to her ear.

Bill was already walking toward the lakeshore, looking like an avian pied piper. A waddling mass of ducks and geese was gathering at his heels. Waterfowl made beelines toward Bill's bright red jacket, swimming over from all corners of the lake. Fluffy brown squirrels appeared as if Bill had called them by name. They skittered down smooth tree trunks and from underneath gnarled tree roots. One grasped a peanut that had fallen out of Bill's pocket, sitting on his haunches to nibble contentedly at his prize.

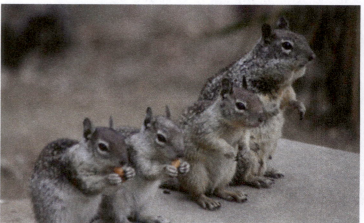

Squirrel friends at Chollas Lake

"Here is my friend, Philip the Goose," Bill said, pointing at the brown-white bird as he sidled up to us. "Hold your hand out flat so that he can get some seed without nipping you." I extended my hand as coached. Philip's long neck extended and recoiled with each thrust of his beak; he pecked with surprising force.

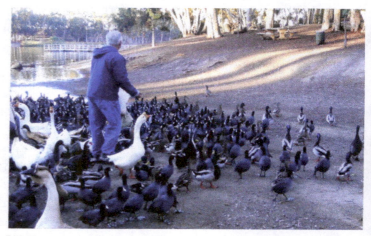

Bill, Feeding the Ducks at Chollas Lake Park

FALLING IN LOVE WITH THE PROCESS: CULTIVATING RESILIENCE IN HEALTH CRISES

"Come here. I want to show you this," Bill beckoned in a hushed tone. We waded through ruffling feathers and webbed feet toward a short dock at the edge of the lake. A brown-flecked duck was huddled against the concrete structure, oddly still. "Look," Bill whispered, pointing underneath the bird's wing.

"Awww," I breathed. Several baby ducks were nestled there, tiny balls of black-and-yellow fluff.

"Ah, and here is Barbara," Bill said, gesturing to a brown goose with a distinct bump on the bridge of her beak. "I named her after the famous Barbara Streisand," Bill winked, smiling as we laughed at his joke.

"How did you start feeding the ducks, Bill?" I asked

"Well, I came down to the lake one day while I was still recovering from my stroke," Bill replied. "There was a mallard—I named him Curly. His beak was all twisted and distorted. He couldn't really eat very well; he looked very thin and hungry. I decided that I would hand-feed him. I came every day, even though it was difficult to drive and walk because of the stroke. Eventually, I started feeding all of the birds. I think it was really important to my recovery," Bill reflected. "They needed me—they were depending on me."

As Patricia and I climbed back into her car, I remember thinking that there was something extremely compelling about this character—Bill Torres—that I had just met. *Yes*, I thought, *there's a book here.*

***

Patricia's chance meeting with Bill Torres at Lake Murray jumpstarted the collaborative relationship behind the stories you are about to read. We sat down with Bill and interviewed him over 20 times. To enlarge our understanding of Bill and his story of recovery and advocacy we reached out to people who knew Bill or were touched by him in some way. Bill offered us the names and contact information for his close friends and for health care providers who worked with him after his stroke. He also put us in touch with other stroke survivors who he worked with during their recovery. In this book, we write to capture what it felt like to meet and speak with the vibrant, engaging people who played such key roles in Bill's life.

Determination, persistence, courage, resilience, strength, and optimism; these are just a few of the words that our interviewees used to describe Bill and his recovery journey. In our time listening to Bill's stories, we have learned that these characteristics didn't just appear after his stroke. These are qualities he developed throughout his lifetime. The stories included in the chapters that follow offer insight about what it takes to cultivate resilience in response to health crises.

But Bill didn't accomplish his recovery alone. The stories offered in this book reveal how crucial it is to have access to a network of support throughout the rehabilitation process. Family members, friends, and caregivers provide us with inspiration, hope, and a reason to keep trying, even when it seems like we are making no progress. As an advocate and a mentor, Bill uses his own story to connect with fellow survivors who feel overwhelmed or disheartened. When he walks into a hospital room and meets a stroke survivor for the first time, he becomes a walking, breathing representation of what recovery can look like.

STRUCTURE OF THE BOOK

We knew from the beginning of our collaboration that Bill's story of recovery and advocacy was significantly interrelated with his life story. This led to our decision to structure the book along two different timelines—the timeline of Bill's early life and the timeline of his life from stroke onward. We alternate between chapters that offer Bill's stories of growing up in San Diego and chapters that provide accounts of Bill's journey of stroke recovery. These two separate storylines come together near the close of the book as we explore Bill's approach to advocacy and mentorship as a stroke survivor.

We have divided the book into three parts. In *Part One: Picking Up the Pieces; Connecting the Dots*, we explore the immediate aftermath of Bill's stroke. We write about the ways in which stigma, depression, and internalized ableism shaped Bill's initially difficult emotional response to stroke but also offer accounts of how his communication with key health care providers reinforced Bill's drive to work on his own rehabilitation. The chapters about his life reveal characteristics he developed as a boy and a young man that contributed to his recovery. In *Part Two: Persisting Through Recovery*, we consider both Bill's capacity to structure his own rehabilitation routine and the ways in which his close network of friends supported him throughout his recovery process. We also see how his career success was fueled by some of the same characteristics that facilitated his recovery. In *Part Three: Communicating as an Advocate*, we explore how Bill transformed his survivor narrative into a tool for advocacy. We outline the strategies Bill used to successfully work with other stroke survivors and also describe the compassion fatigue that can accompany this kind of communicative labor. At the end of each part, we connect to literature from health communication and other relevant academic fields to describe the communication lessons apparent in Bill's life story. But first, we begin at the beginning—the day of Bill's stroke.

REFERENCE

Levine, P. G. (2013). *Stronger after stroke: Your recovery roadmap to recovery* (2nd ed.). New York, NY: demosHEALTH.

PART 1

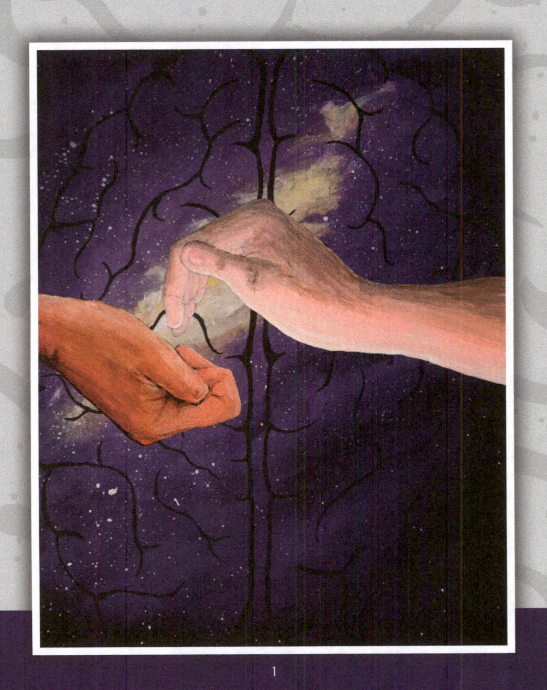

"Illness is the night-side of life, a more onerous citizenship. Everyone who is born holds dual citizenship, in the kingdom of the well and in the kingdom of the sick. Although we all prefer to use only the good passport, sooner or later each of us is obliged, at least for a spell, to identify ourselves as citizens of that other place" (p. 3).

—Susan Sontag (1978), *Illness as Metaphor*

"To name an illness is to describe a certain condition of suffering—a literary act before it becomes a medical one. A patient, long before he [or she] becomes the subject of medical scrutiny, is, at first, simply a storyteller, a narrator of suffering—a traveler who has visited the kingdom of the ill. To relieve an illness, one must begin, then by unburdening the story" (p. 46).

—Siddhartha Mukherjee (2010),
The Emperor of all Maladies: A Biography of Cancer

In Chapter 1 of *Part One: Picking up the Pieces; Connecting the Dots*, we meet Bill Torres at a turning point moment in his life when he experienced a paralyzing stroke. We find ourselves inside his story and discover the sense he is trying to make of this devastating moment. In Chapter 2, we shift gears to discover where and when Bill was born and how some of his earliest experiences may in some way have contributed to his ability to become a resilient stroke survivor. By Chapter 3, we begin to see the ways in which the stroke has affected Bill's body and the effort he must exert to engage in simple tasks that many of us take for granted. Stroke has shattered Bill's life, leaving him with the painful task of picking up the pieces. Chapter 4 continues the story of Bill's life, following his youthful quest to find love and adventure, detailing the losses he faces along his journeys. In Chapter 5, we begin to see that the road to recovery is rocky, not only because of the length of time it takes to gain back simple functioning but also because of the inevitable depression that threatens Bill's capacity to persist. Finally, Chapter 6 expands Bill's story to reveal how he has always been on the move, getting bored, and looking for new experiences, a characteristic that served him well as he continued to connect the dots in his recovery.

CHAPTER 1

"The day prior to the stroke I was playing paddleball with Charlie Brumfield. He ran me all over the court," Bill recounts. We're seated in a quiet corner of Lake Murray Café, the local diner Bill often frequents after his morning visits with the ducks. Bill is sporting a full, gray, neatly trimmed beard—something Patricia has not seen on him before.

"I went over to my mother's house the next morning to take her to breakfast," Bill continues. "I was sitting down for a nice game of crossword puzzle, and I couldn't make an A. I tried, but my hand would just go right off the paper. So, I stood up and said, 'What the hell is coming over me?'

Mom asked me, 'Where are we going to go for breakfast?'

I went to say, 'The French pastries shop, which is your favorite.' Instead, I went 'blah, blah, blah'—the words wouldn't come out.

So, I went in the other room and was testing—'one-two, one-two'—and then my voice came back. I figured, *something is wrong*. I couldn't write, I couldn't speak. *Something is wrong*. I said, 'Mom, I'm going to call up Sheila. I want her to come. I'm going to run an errand with her and then I will be right back.' I didn't want to frighten her.

So, I called up my friend Sheila and I said, 'Sheila, come and get me. I think I had a stroke.'"

MEETING SHEILA

"I love Florida." Sheila's eyes gleam when Sarah tells her that she lives and works near Orlando now. She looks younger than the 60 she is about to be in two weeks, especially when her smile transforms her angular face, crinkling her button nose. The three of us settle into the cold metal chairs at Starbucks, a bit of relief on this warm, windy San Diego day. We would have preferred to sit inside because of all the traffic noise outside, but there isn't a table or chair to spare in the crowded cafe.

Interview contributed by Sheila Holdway. Copyright © Kendall Hunt Publishing Company.

We sit for a few seconds in silence; having heard so much about each other through Bill, we feel like old friends getting together to chat about anything, everything.

"I'm excited to finally be talking with you," Sarah says.

"Yes," Patricia laughs, "because Bill's been like, 'Let's get started on this book. I could die here!"

"I know. He keeps saying that," Sarah agrees, rolling her eyes in mock frustration. "We're like, '*Bill*'!"

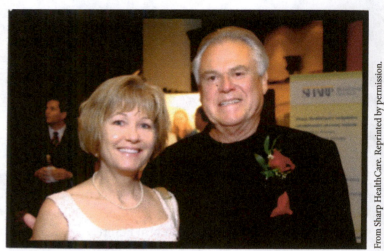

Sheila and Bill at Sharp's Victories of Spirit Banquet

"Let me tell you, I call him every day," Sheila says. "And if he doesn't answer the phone, I'm like, 'You're dead. Call me back because I don't know what to do.' And then a couple of times he hasn't called back, and I've gotten in my car and driven over to see if his car is there."

CALLING THE AMBULANCE

"I sat out on the porch, and Sheila comes flying up," Bill continues. "I went to get up. I just fell over around the railing and I was completely paralyzed. I couldn't move anything. All I could do was blink my eyes and I was trying to tell her one for no and two for yes or whatever. And she said, 'Are you okay?'"

***

"He tells it a little different," Sheila says, "I'm like, 'No, that's not what happened. What are you talking about?'" She leans against the cold metal back of her Starbucks' chair, launching into her version of events. "At the time of the stroke, Bill was staying at home with his mom all the time and she was living in a trailer," Sheila explains. "Bill always lived in really nice places, but he wanted to make sure she was okay because she was 90-something. She was in good health, but she was alone and he was concerned about her. He told me, 'I'll just stay with my mom for a while because I don't know how much longer I'm going to have her.'"

Bill and his mom got along great, but sometimes you just need space. So sometimes on Sundays he would come over to my house and watch football, which I don't do. I would clean my house and do stuff, and then he'd tell me what the score was. His mom would have been switching the TV channels back and forth, so I just let him sit there and watch the game. On the day of the stroke, he was going to come over to watch the game. So, I called him and said, 'OK, do you want anything to eat or have lunch or whatever?'

He goes, 'No, I'm fine. The weirdest thing happened to me. I was doing the crossword puzzle and the pencil dropped out of my hand.'

At first, I didn't think anything of it. I go, 'What?'

And he goes, 'Yes, it just fell right out of my hand.'

And I go, 'That's weird.'

He said, 'I picked it up and finished the puzzle.'

And I said, 'Good. When are you going to be here?'

He said, 'I'll probably be there in a half hour or 45 minutes.' A half hour and 45 minutes went by and he wasn't there, and that was very unlike him because he is very on time. So I called him, and it was as if, when I was talking to him, he wasn't making sense. He sounded weird, so I asked him 'Where are you?'

He said something like, 'Well, I haven't taken a shower yet.'

And I'm like, 'What the heck?' That was definitely not like him. I go, 'You haven't taken a shower yet?'

He goes, 'No. I'm going to get into the shower here in a minute. I should be there in about half hour.'

I hang up the phone and go, 'That was odd.' Then a half hour went by and I called him because he wasn't there, and he didn't sound right to me. He's still there at his mom's, and he hadn't even taken a shower yet. I didn't know what to think.

He was like, 'I'm going to be there soon.'

I said, 'You stay where you are. I'm going to come to you.' I hadn't even been to his mom's trailer park, but I knew where it was. I drove over there, and as I'm pulling up and getting out of my car, he's coming out. He's sort of waving at me, but he's dragging his foot and his arm.

I'm like, 'Oh my God.' I reach back into my car and get my phone, and I dial 911.

He's like, 'What are you doing?'

I said, 'You've had a stroke.'

He's like, 'What?'

I'm like, 'You've had a stroke. You have to sit down or something. Look at your arm. Something's wrong. Something's wrong. I think you've had a stroke.' Then, I called the ambulance."

**

"But I knew that there was something wrong right away," Bill tells us, "And most people don't. You know most people—especially guys—have this little macho-ism. A lot people just go to bed and say, 'I'll wake up in the morning and I'll be okay.' They don't want to go to the doctor.

All I know is that I didn't want to scare my mother, so that's when I called my friend Sheila. There was no pain involved whatsoever. Nothing. All I could think of at that moment was, 'What's going to happen to my mom?' I was thinking she can't lose me because she already lost my sister. I've got to live through this. That's all I remember, and then I passed out. I went unconscious."

THE WAITING NEVER ENDS

"I sat out in the waiting room for a little while, because I told his mom I would let her know what's going on," Sheila says. "Finally, I'm sitting there for an hour or whatever, and then I went and knocked on the door and said, 'Do you know …? My friend is in there. Can anybody tell me …?'

They go, 'Do you want to go in with him?'

I'm like, 'I didn't know I could.' They let me go in and he was lying there. By then he knew he'd had a stroke, and he could feel it coming. He kept having them on that table.

The hospital staff kept asking me, 'How long has he been showing signs of a stroke?'

I'm like, 'You could have asked me this a long time ago,' because they only want to give that medicine to you if it's within so many hours of having a stroke.[1]

---

1. "Alteplase IV r-tPA is given through an IV in the arm, also known tPA, and works by dissolving the clot and improving blood flow to the part of the brain being deprived of blood flow …. [It] needs to be used within three hours of having a stroke or up to 4.5 hours in certain eligible patients. Many people miss this key brain-saving treatment because they don't arrive at the hospital in time for alteplase treatment, which is why it's so important to identify a stroke and seek treatment immediately for the best possible chance at a full recovery" (American Stroke Association, 2018).

FALLING IN LOVE WITH THE PROCESS: CULTIVATING RESILIENCE IN HEALTH CRISES

I don't know if they gave him that medicine or not, but then he'd say, 'It's going to happen in a minute. I can feel it.' He'd go out a little bit, and then he'd come to. He'd say, 'You see that?' And then I'd go, 'Yes, I saw that.' He knew right when it was happening.

***

"The paramedics took me to Sharp," Bill recalls. "I kept passing out. I had like 12 strokes. I'd come to and I'd say, 'I feel great … oh no, here it comes.' I kept coming in and out of them. I remember when they were wheeling me down to emergency, they were all panicking. My voice comes back and I'm trying to say, 'Hey, don't panic. I had a stroke. Take it easy. I'll be good, I just had a stroke.'

I heard the doctor saying, 'Call the cardiologist, his heart rate is 38 beats per minute. We're going to have to put a pacemaker in.[2] I came to. I heard what she was saying and my voice came back. I actually said, 'No. don't do that. Check it, that's my natural heart rate, check it again.' So, it was a minor miracle that my voice came back and they didn't put in a pacemaker. When your heart rate is below 50, and if you're unconscious, I guess they put a pacemaker in you.

Then I remember them wheeling me down to Rehab. The way from ICU to Rehab was down a long, temporary tunnel. When I opened my eyes, the tunnel was dimly lit. I was confused and scared. I was taken to a room in the stroke ward, put in bed, and left alone. I thought, *What's next?*"

***

"They said, 'We're going to transfer him over to the other part of the hospital,'" Sheila continues. "So, I told his mom I'd check on him. I took his Rolex and I said, 'Let me have your phone and your watch. I'm going to take them with me.' I took those two things and then started calling people and telling them that he'd had a stroke, and he was at Sharp Hospital, but that I didn't know any news. I didn't know anything yet, I was just letting them know—I could look through his phone contacts and let some people know. Bill didn't know I did that. Three years later, he kept talking about, 'I heard all those people visited me in the hospital, and I didn't even know how they knew I was there.' I'm like, 'I called them. I called them. I'm the one who took your phone and called them.'

'No, I don't remember that,' he would say. I was calling people, and I didn't even get any credit. I said to Bill, 'What the hell? You mean all this time I didn't get any credit for that? You just thought people were miraculously showing up at the hospital, like the universe told them?'"

***

2. A normal resting heart rate for adults ranges from 60 to 100 beats per minute. Generally, a lower heart rate at rest implies more efficient heart function and better cardiovascular fitness. For example, a well-trained athlete might have a normal resting heart rate closer to 40 beats per minute. https://www.mayoclinic.org/healthy-lifestyle/fitness/expert-answers/heart-rate/faq-20057979

"They did an X-ray of my brain and then an MRI," Bill remembers. "Then, they had me swallow some water because they wanted to see if my epiglottis was working. If it's not working, they have to feed you through your stomach because you're choking. I didn't want to be fed through my stomach. I sipped some water, cheering for my epiglottis to function. I lucked out; it worked. Now, I only had to cope with a useless right side."

CLOSING REFLECTIONS

Stroke is the second leading cause of death worldwide and the fifth leading cause of death in the United States (Wallace, 2019). A stroke occurs "when a blood vessel that carries oxygen and nutrients to the brain is either blocked by a clot or bursts (or ruptures). When that happens, part of the brain cannot get the blood (and oxygen) it needs, so it and brain cells die" (American Stroke Association, 2018). Only 10% of victims of stroke make a complete recovery and thus 90 % live with the disabilities caused by stroke (National Stroke Association, 2018). What is most alarming is that between the years 2000 and 2010, there was a 44% increase in stroke for people ages 25 to 44 (Ramirez et al., 2016). No matter what the age of the stroke victim, a stroke can cause a range of disabilities, including permanent loss of speech, movement, and memory (National Stroke Association, 2018).

Research reveals that those survivors who have the most success at recovery begin and sustain their rehabilitation just a few days after the stroke. The stroke-related phrase that is often repeated is time-loss is brain-loss. "In each minute, 1.9 million neurons . . . are destroyed" (Saver, 2006, p. 263), which increases the risk of disability or death. The National Stroke Association has established the campaign Act FAST:

Use FAST to Remember the Warning Signs of a Stroke

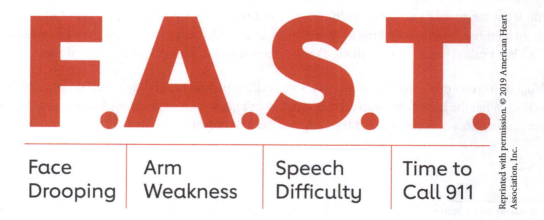

Reprinted with permission. © 2019 American Heart Association, Inc.

This is especially a liability for young people who delay seeking treatment because they do not recognize these symptoms or because they believe that strokes only happen to the elderly (Wallace, 2017).

Unfortunately, the emotional and physical struggles survivors face after the stroke often result in depression and the inability to take the action needed for recovery. Too often, stroke survivors experience a negative sense of self and, as a result, reduce their social activity and settle on a restricted future because of their physical disabilities (Ellis-Hill & Horn, 2000). In fact, research reveals that one out of eight stroke survivors considers suicide (Bartoli et al., 2017). Even one year after the stroke, survivors experience risk factors such as depression, disability, insomnia, suicidal ideation, and stroke recurrence (Yang et al., 2017). Thus, it is essential to consider the meaning of the stroke within the life of each individual in order for providers, family members, and friends to play a significant role in stroke survivors' recovery.

We close this chapter with questions to consider that this book will attempt to answer. First, are there characteristics that people develop at a young age or throughout their lifetime that contribute to their resiliency in recovery? Second, what roles do supportive relationships with family and friends play in survivors' recovery from stroke? Third, how does a stroke survivor's engagement in advocacy—helping others recover from stroke—strengthen the survivor's resiliency and recovery? Fourth, how does listening and being listened to contribute to a stroke survivors' resiliency, recovery, and advocacy?

This chapter is just the beginning of our journey through Bill's storied life. The chapters that follow alternate between his life story and his recovery and advocacy stories. In the next chapter, we take a look back over 80 years ago, when Bill was born. We discover what his life was like growing up in San Diego, the paths he followed as a young man, and consider how experiences from his earlier years may have shaped the way he responded to the devastation of his stroke.

REFERENCES

American Stroke Association. (2018). *About stroke.* Retrieved from https://www.strokeassociation.org/STROKEORG/AboutStroke/About-Stroke_UCM_308529_SubHomePage.jsp

Bartoli, F., Pompili, M., Lillia, N., Crocamo, C., Salemi, G., Clerici, M., & Carra, G. (2017). Rates and correlates of suicidal ideation among stroke survivors: A meta-analysis. *Journal of Neurological Neurosurgical Psychiatry, 88*, 498–504.

Ellis-Hill, C. S., & Horn, S. (2000). Change in identity and self concept: A new theoretical approach to recovery following a stroke. *Clinical Rehabilitation, 14*, 279-287.

National Stroke Association. (2018). *Stroke recovery.* Retrieved from http://www.stroke.org/we-can-help/survivors/stroke-recovery

Ramirez, L., Kim-Tenser, M. A., Sanossian, N., Cen, S., Wen, G., He, S,, Mack, W. J., Towfighi, A. (2016). Trends in acute ischemic stroke hospitalizations in the United States. *Journal of American Heart Association, 5* (5), doi: 10.1161/JAHA.116.003233.

Saver, J. L. (2006). Time is brain--Quantified. *Stroke, 37*, 263-266. doi.org/10.1161/01

Wallace, J. B. (2016, May 11). Researchers document troubling rise in strokes in young adults, starting at age 25.

Wallace, J. B. (2017, December 5). Different strokes. *The San Diego Union-Tribune*, E 1-2.

Yang, Y., Shi, Y. Z., Zhang, N., Wang, S., Ungvari, G. S., Ng, C. H., … Xiang, Y. T. (2017). Suicidal ideation at 1-year post-stroke: A nationwide survey in China. *General Hospital Psychiatry, 44*, 38–42.

CHAPTER 2

"There used to be a streetcar running down here to the beach," Bill says, pointing at what is now a crowded intersection on the Point Loma peninsula of San Diego. He keeps up a running commentary from the backseat of Patricia's Honda CRV, entertaining us on our journey back from an interview with some of his oldest friends. Driving around San Diego with Bill is like viewing the city through the sepia frames of an old film strip; memories from his life overlay the contours of current-day neighborhoods, tinting them with nostalgia.

We've timed our ride home just right; the setting sun slips slowly beneath the Pacific Ocean, bathing us in the pink rays of the fading day as we round the curve of Sunset Cliffs. Tourists and locals stroll along the crumbling sandstone edges, drinking in views of both the ocean and the impressive cliff-side mansions. Many of these homes are familiar to Bill. We've just passed a boxy pink stucco estate with gaudy white columns—a place where Bill used to party as a young man.

"My Uncle Denny was a streetcar driver," Bill continues. "When I was five, he used to take me for rides along the coast. I would point toward La Jolla and ask, 'who lives over there?' 'Only crazy people,' he'd say. Back then, it was all sand dunes."

We laugh together at this memory, trying to imagine a time when hoity-toity La Jolla was free of its trendy shops and the sleek, modern glass-and-steel houses of the superrich. Sarah turns to look back at Bill from the passenger seat.

"Would you tell us a little more about your childhood?"

***

John William Torres was born September 6, 1935, delivered by his father, Joe, and his grandfather in his parents' bedroom. His mom was named Louise, but everyone called her "Babe." When her son was born, Babe gave him a nickname as well—Billy. "Billy" was born in Old Town, San Diego. As the historic heart of the original Spanish settlement, Old Town has since been transformed into a tourist destination with museums, missions, and Mexican restaurants. Its evolution was shaped by many of the same forces that influenced Bill's life—the Great Depression, World War II, Mexican immigration, and the desire to shift out of poverty and toward prosperity.

A CHILD OF THE GREAT DEPRESSION

At the time of Bill's birth, San Diego's economy, like most U.S. cities, had slowed with the country's Great Depression. While depressions in the economy were happening every ten years, The Great Depression was considered the most devastating in terms of its length and depth. Between the stock market crash of 1929 and the beginning of World War II in 1941, "fifteen million Americans, a quarter of the work force, lost their jobs. Millions more lost their homes, farms, businesses, and life savings" (DiGiorolamo, 2018, para. 1). A common saying during that era was "use it up, wear it out, make it do, or go without" (Cavanaugh & Walsh, 2009, para. 1).

Looking back, Bill describes growing up in the Great Depression as a lean time. "When I was six or seven years old, we were very poor," he recalls. "My dad would go up to the grocery store and get all the bad potatoes that were thrown out. I remember him cutting away the bad parts and keeping the good parts. I used to go up to ask the butcher for bones for the dog, and the butcher knew we were poor. The butcher knew everyone in the area. It was a little store in Old Town. He'd always give me bones with some meat on them so my mother would make soup. I remember that. I remember that vividly."

"I can remember going to the store just to buy a loaf of bread from Mr. Helman. I went and got a loaf of bread. I put down a dime. He says, 'Oh, Billy, you're going to have to tell your mom she owes me a penny because the bread went up two cents.' It was nine cents a loaf; it was now 11 cents. I remember him taking out the little pad—those green pads that give you the receipt—and clipping a note that says, 'Babe owes one penny.'"

Despite these memories of poverty, Bill didn't realize that he was poor as a child—mostly because of his parents' ingenuity. "Kids in the neighborhood always used to like to come to my house because my mother was creative with potatoes," Bill remembers. "Mashed potatoes, scalloped potatoes, boiled potatoes, French fries, shredded potatoes. The other kids didn't get that at home. They thought it was a treat, and I'm saying, 'Hey, this is great.' We ate potatoes."

One school of thought about the impact of the Great Depression on children is that this devastating decade strengthened children's character, creating America's "greatest generation" of the World War II era. Bill's first grade report card reveals a strength of character that bore out for the rest of his life. Mrs. Devlin, his teacher, wrote, "Billy is a very good worker. He is always ready to help others. He likes to read, and often reads extra stories."

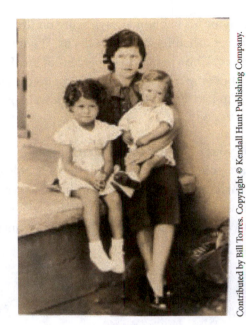

Gloria, Mom, Billy (age 1)

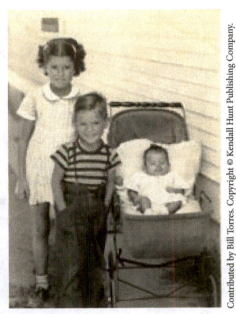

Gloria, Billy (age 6), Joanne

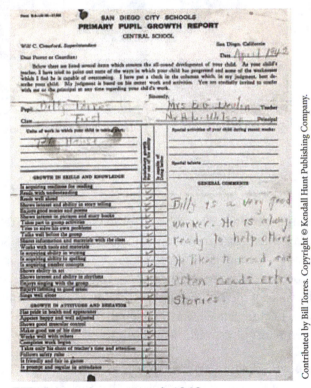

Bill's first grade report card, 1942

Bill credits his mother and father for his work ethic, and for his habit of always being on time. "My mother and father never missed a day of work. They never called in sick," Bill tells us. "I got that in my brain—that you show up. To me, as Woody Allen said, 'Showing up is 80 percent of life. Sometimes it's easier to hide home in bed. I've done both.'" Bill emphasizes, "if you tell me to do something, I will do it. If you tell me to be here at 9 o'clock, I'm here at five to nine. You can walk out the door and I will be standing there."

For Bill, "showing up" also means committing to doing your best. "My mother taught me, if you are going to do something, do it right," Bill says. "If you are going to dig a hole, dig the best hole possible. If you're going to wax the floor, wax the floor. Whatever you do, whatever your job is, you do it to the best of your ability, be proud of it. I carry that with me." Clearly, Bill's parents had a strong influence on his character. Being a child during World War II may have also played a significant role in shaping his personality.

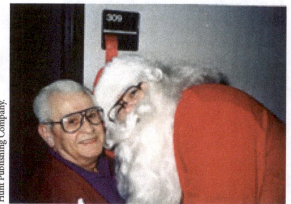

Bill's father, Joe Torres, age 86 (and Santa!)

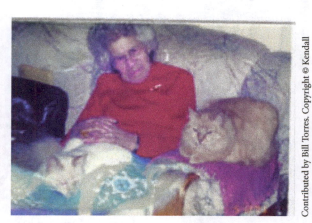

Bill's mother, "Babe" Torres (with cats!)

A CHILD OF WAR

Bill had just turned six in September 1941 when World War II began. Yet, he vividly remembers that fateful December day when America finally joined the fray. "It was Sunday," Bill recalls. "I'm walking [toward] University Avenue and a big truck goes by throwing these papers—big stacks of papers—and the paper boys were grabbing the papers saying, 'Extra! Extra! World War II, Pearl Harbor bombed!'" In the wake of the Japanese attack, San Diegans were convinced that their bayside military base would be the next target. Viewed through the lens of Bill's memories, modern-day San Diego is speckled with remnants of its wartime preparations.

As we drive together through Mission Valley traffic, Bill points to a white, turreted building perched high above us on the edge of the canyon. He explains that the fortress-like structure, now likely a million-dollar home, once housed a massive gun, aimed to shoot down enemy bombers as they entered the mouth of the valley.

Bill's childhood recollections are similarly marked by the exigencies of wartime defense. "In front of our house, we had a 55-gallon [kerosene] drum with a smokestack," Bill recounts, sharing a picture of his family in front of his childhood home. A barrage balloon floats in the background. It is one craft in a flotilla that defended San Diego against aircraft attack using cables that posed a collision hazard for enemy planes.

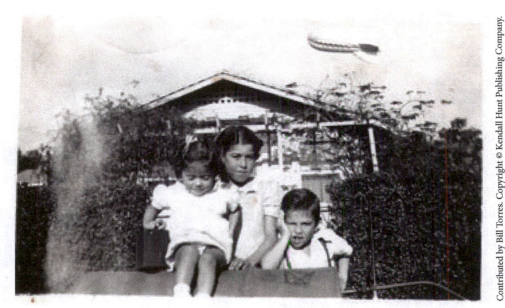

Joanne, Gloria, and Bill (age 5) leaning on the kerosene drum in front of their house

"Sometimes, we would have air raid drills," Bill recalls. "You'd hear the sirens, and then you had to go into your house and block out your windows with black shades. Then they'd light that kerosene on fire and send up a smokescreen so all of Old Town would be flooded with smoke and hidden from any overhead planes. Then the soldiers would be running through your house, through your yard. They'd all have guns. They had a military tank out on San Diego Avenue, and they'd let us go inside. The soldiers were real nice." Some of those soldiers were his friends' older brothers, drafted into battle at age 18. One lucky neighborhood teen was shot just as his landing craft beached at the battle of Iwo Jima. He returned to San Diego with a few injuries and a large, shiny medal—proudly displaying it for Bill and his friends.

Of course, Bill's father couldn't join the war effort because he had three young children. Instead, he and Babe worked 12-hour shifts at Consolidated Aircraft Corporation. Headquartered in Buffalo, New York, Consolidated opened its West Coast Convair assembly plant to build B24 bombers and

PBY Catalina seaplanes. The huge factory was carefully camouflaged against air attacks. "If you were to fly over it, you would see they had cars—just the outer frame of the cars—sitting on top," Bill remembers. "If the bombers had come over, they'd say, 'That's just a road.'"

After the war, everyone at Consolidated got laid off. Bill's father became a commercial tuna fisherman. He would be gone one to three months at a time. Perhaps it was that time away—and his father's drinking—that laid the seeds for Bill's parents' divorce.

A CHILD OF DIVORCE

Bill's father's alcoholism drove a wedge between his parents, eventually contributing to their decision to divorce when Bill was in ninth grade. What made the divorce even more difficult for Bill's mother was the rejection she experienced from her six sisters, who objected to divorce because of their staunch Catholic faith. "They didn't talk to her for five, six years, some ten years," Bill tells us. "It was hard on her because they were close. They grew up in San Diego, seven daughters and mother and father in a two-bedroom house—the same house that I grew up in Old Town." Over the years, the sisters reunited. Pictured here are all seven sisters, from the oldest to the youngest.

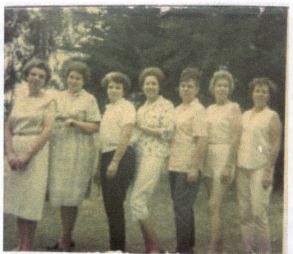

Vera, Mary, Jenny, Belle, Stella, Bill's Mom Babe, and Dally

The struggle with poverty continued in their family of four—Bill and his mom, his older sister, Gloria, and his little sister, Joanne. As a single mother, Babe managed to scrape together US$4,000 to buy a small house in Golden Hill. Bill still remembers dinner with his mother on the first night in their new home. "There was nothing in the house for dinner except two cans that didn't have labels on them. I was the man of the house. I got to choose what can we'd eat for dinner that night. I said, 'I'll take this can here.' We opened it up—I'll never forget. In fact, I had some today. They were beets. We ate beets for dinner. We thought that was great. We didn't think anything of it." Bill's account is filtered through his optimistic approach to life. "You don't think you're poor," he elaborates. "I had two pairs of shoes. I had some jeans, some T-shirts. I was happy. Never had a suit or anything like that for dances, going into the 12th grade."

It's a credit to Babe that her three children didn't think of themselves as poor or resent doing without enough. Yet, these experiences of poverty intersected with subtle and overt racism that the family experienced as a result of their Mexican roots.

A CHILD OF IMMIGRANTS

In 1935, the same year that Bill was born, San Diego officials attempted to remedy the ills of the Great Depression and boost tourism by hosting the California Pacific International Exposition in the city's famed Balboa Park. Several new buildings were constructed for this purpose, including the Globe Theater—a replica of William Shakespeare's renowned London stage. The round, brown stucco building, with its dark wooden beams and leaded windows stands in stark contrast to the neighboring, equally iconic structure—the California Tower. Built in 1915 for the California-Panama Exposition, the California Tower boasts the ornate façade of a Spanish Colonial church, as well as a massive dome decorated with cobalt-and-white-checked tiles and golden mosaic stars reminiscent of the Church of Santa Prisca and San Sebastián in Taxco, Mexico.

This English–Spanish–Mexican mashup echoes Bill's own ancestry. Bill's grandparents on his father's side were from Mexico—Ensenada and Mazatlán. They immigrated to San Diego around 1910, and Bill's father was born and raised in San Diego. On his mother's side, Bill's grandfather was English and very wealthy, and his grandmother was from Ensenada. His grandfather's family disowned him for marrying a Mexican woman.

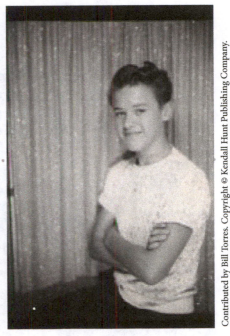

Bill, age 16

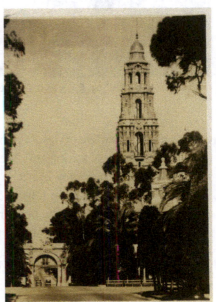

Balboa Park's California Tower in the early 1900s

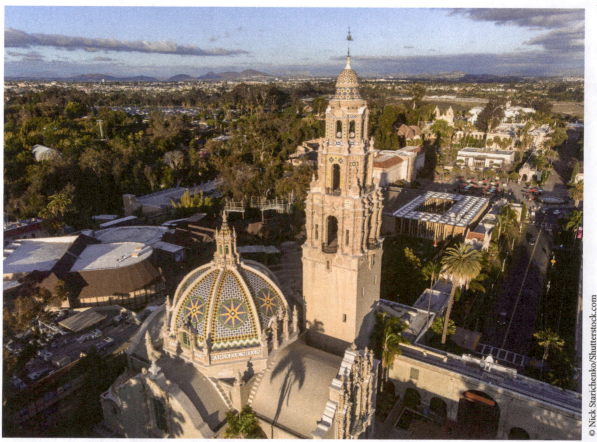

Overall view of Balboa Park and the California Tower in San Diego, California.

Growing up in San Diego near the border of Mexico translated to another struggle for Bill's family, given the presence of strong anti-Mexican prejudice at the time. We know that the Great Depression was especially difficult for Mexican immigrants. They constantly faced the threat of deportation, along with the shortages in jobs and food that affected the entire population. Discrimination was especially apparent along the borderland between San Diego, CA and Tijuana, Mexico. DiGiorolamo (2018) provided this account of the Mexican experience in 1930s America:

> As unemployment swept the U.S., hostility to immigrant workers grew, and the government began a program of repatriating immigrants to Mexico. Immigrants were offered free train rides to Mexico, and some went voluntarily, but many were either tricked or coerced into repatriation, and some U.S. citizens were deported simply on suspicion of being Mexican. All in all, hundreds of thousands of Mexican immigrants, especially farmworkers, were sent out of the country during the 1930s—many of them the same workers who had been eagerly recruited a decade before. (para. 1)

Bill tells us that this discrimination found its way directly into his family for both his father and mother. For example, Bill's dad told him that in the early 1900s, Mexicans and African Americans were restricted to one day of swimming—Tuesdays—in the local Morley Pool in Balboa Park. Bill explains, "On Tuesday night, that's when they cleaned the pool, chlorinated it for the White people for the next day. So, on Tuesdays Blacks and Mexicans could go swimming."

Bill's mom described discrimination that her sisters faced. Two of her sisters could not have children and wanted to adopt but were not permitted to. As Bill explains, "even though their maiden name was Williams, you had to put mother and father, and if your mother was Mexican or father was Mexican you weren't allowed to adopt."

Unlike his father and mother, Bill can't remember situations where he was discriminated against directly, in his view because he was light-skinned and no one really perceived of him as Mexican. The only occasion that stands out in his mind happened when he was 17. His mother's boyfriend invited him along on a drive to the small town of Gothenburg, Nebraska, to pick up his son and bring him back to San Diego. Once they arrived, about 20 of the town's children came to see Bill because they'd never seen a Mexican in person.

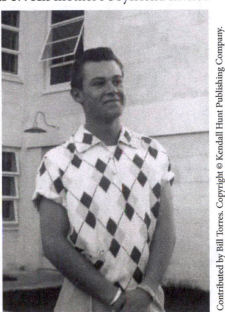

Contributed by Bill Torres. Copyright © Kendall Hunt Publishing Company.

"'They said, 'Well, you don't look Mexican.'

I said, 'What does a Mexican look like?'

They said, 'They wear a big sombrero and they sit next to a cactus and sleep.'"

Bill was shocked by the idea that anyone would believe such blatantly stereotypical caricatures of Mexican culture. As he entered adulthood, however, Bill began to realize that his Californian upbringing had shielded him from the true depth of racism in 1950s America.

Bill, age 17

A YOUNG ADULT IN A SEGREGATED UNITED STATES

Bill graduated from San Diego High School in 1953, the same high school his father attended. After graduation, Bill joined the U.S. Air Force and served in Sacramento from 1954 to 1958. When he was 19, Bill traveled to New Orleans with his fellow service members. His stories from the trip capture clear examples of the segregation and discrimination that Black Americans faced at that time.

"I was shocked to see how Blacks got off of the sidewalk when you were walking toward them," Bill recalls. "They got off and let you go by. In the rest rooms, they had Colored restrooms and White restrooms. There was a Colored waiting room when we had to take a bus, and a White waiting room. We decided to take a bus just to cruise Bourbon Street. When we got on the bus and sat in the back, the bus driver stopped.

He says, 'You guys can't sit back there.'

I say, 'What do you mean we can't sit back here?'

'That's for niggers only.'

'Wait, what?'

'Get your ass up here and sit up here where you belong.' We had to get up and sit up in the front. My friend and I (he was from LA and I was from San Diego) had never seen this before."

Bill was particularly struck by the discrimination experienced by Black members of the air force, who were integrated in the service but often received the worst assignments. While he was friendly with his Black compatriots, segregation made socializing difficult. Bill relayed a series of challenges he faced when he attempted to go off base and see a movie with his friend, Washington:

"We jumped in the cab and the driver says, 'You know you can't go off base with that black guy there.'

I said, 'What?'

He says, 'I will drop you off at the gate because I can't take you.'

We get out and I see air police at the gate. I said, 'Why can't this guy go with us? We're going downtown.'

He says, 'Either he walks in front of you, or behind you. Not together, or you're in trouble.'

Washington says, 'Come on, let's go to the movies.' He walks behind me. So, we get to the movies, we pay for the movie, and the ticket taker says, 'Colored people upstairs, White people downstairs.'

Bill was uncomfortable with the racism he witnessed, so he found as many ways as he could to resist it—with questions, with his affable personality, and with his trademark sarcasm.

"I remember going over and drinking at the fountain in the bus station," Bill recalls. "I go over to the fountain labeled *Colored* and drink out of it.

One of the workers said, 'Hey, you can't drink out of it.'

'Well this is wrong,' I said, 'This is supposed to be *colored* water and it's the same color as that water over there for the White fountain.'"

Perhaps it was these experiences of injustice and ignorance that inspired Bill's initial career choice: teaching.

THE START OF A CAREER, THE BIRTH OF A FRIENDSHIP

After his honorable discharge from the air force, Bill attended one semester of college at Sacramento Junior college. Bill would tell you that he is the kind of person who always has to start something new and take it to fulfillment. When he met Dick Kirby in junior college and learned that Dick flew planes, he asked him to teach him how to fly. So, Bill took lessons, learned how to fly, and earned his flying license by 1963. After Junior College, he moved back to San Diego and graduated with a BA in Education at San Diego State University. He earned his teaching credential and began teaching in San Diego City Schools. He also began taking night graduate seminars at San Diego State University.

One especially impactful college course was the Minority Group Relations seminar Bill took in 1962, taught by Professor Tom Gillette. In our interview with Tom, this is how he described their relationship: "Bill was a student in the class. He is almost naturally open to friendships. He and I became friends in the class and every Friday evening, or afternoon, he would meet with his fellow teachers from around the schools where he was teaching. He invited me to come have a drink with them, and so I did."

Of course, Bill's version of the story is a bit more colorful: "That Friday, the party is going on. I wasn't paying attention to whether Tom came in or not," Bill remembers. "Anyway, he walks in and he had been getting certified to be a scuba diver. He still had his wet suit on, and he comes in and says, 'You got anything to drink?'

I say, 'Got some beer, milk, whiskey whatever you like.'

'Oh, milk.'

'Help yourself.'

'I remember him opening the refrigerator door,'" Bill says with a grin, "I always thought it was rude of him to drink out of the carton." That swig of milk started a friendship that would last over 45 years—one that would be a key resource for Bill as he faced the daunting task of recovering from his stroke.

CLOSING REFLECTIONS

Bill's resilience through the Great Depression, the fallout from World War II, his father's alcoholism, his parent's divorce, and being the "man of the house" for his single mother may have, in part, created a foundation for his persistence and strength to accomplish a complete recovery from his stroke. His success post-stroke may have something to do with how both of Bill's parents had a good sense of humor; being silly and laughing were part of everyday life, with both his parents, even after they divorced. Bill sees his sense of humor as what has carried him through any challenge, including his recovery from the stroke. As we move through the stories of Bill's life and his recovery, there is more to learn, not only about his personality but about the creative strategies he utilized to make a full recovery.

What does it feel like to have a stroke? What goes through your mind when you can't form the words to tell people the confusion you are feeling or the ways your body is not functioning in ways you have taken for granted? The next chapter explores Bill's process of waking up from the stroke, not only from his own perspective but from the perspective of a few of the health care providers who vividly remember caring for Bill over ten years ago.

REFERENCES

Cavanaugh, M., & Walsh, N. (2009, August 30). *Life in the 1930s in San Diego*. Retrieved from http://www.kpbs.org/news/2009/aug/20/life-1930s-san-diego/

DiGiorolamo, V. (2018). Depression and the struggle for survival. Growing up in down times: Children of the Great Depression. *HERB: Resources for Teachers*. Retrieved from https://herb.ashp.cuny.edu/items/show/525

CHAPTER 3

Parking karma leads us to a spot near the entrance to Sharp Memorial Hospital. It's a crisp, bright, summer day and we are excited to interview Susan Martinez, the nurse who cared for Bill when he was admitted after his stroke. We chat about how Bill calls Susan his "angel" as we pass through the electronic front door. At the information desk, we learn that we can find Susan at a nearby nurse's station. Just as we arrive there, the emergency doors close behind us. There is a flurry of activity as people respond to a seemingly routine emergency drill. We stand awkwardly for a moment, trying to decide the best time to interrupt politely to ask for Susan, when she appears, looking just like a photo we've seen from so many years ago—wavy blond hair and sunny smile.

"Are you here to interview me about Bill Torres? Why don't we head out to the courtyard, where there's a bit of calm in this chaos?"

We follow her down a short hall and out into the sunshiny day to sit around a concrete table with built-in concrete benches. After we each offer a brief bio of ourselves, Patricia explains, "What we'd like to do is just ask a set of questions about your experience with Bill. We really want to explore his stroke and recovery experience."

"Yes," Sarah elaborates. "It's always helpful for us to start with you telling us about your role here at Sharp."

"OK. I'm a nursing assistant. I've been a nursing assistant for several years. I do direct hands-on care with the patients and I'm also responsible for their activities. I've been here, at this particular facility, for 15 years."

"This is where Bill came after his stroke, right?" Patricia inserts.

"Yes," Susan replies, looking beyond us as if she is picturing a younger Bill standing there. "I can remember Bill so well because we had several moments together in the beginning, where I tried to pull him out of a depression."

Interview contributed by Susan Martinez. Copyright © Kendall Hunt Publishing Company.

Bill describes waking up from the stroke, not as one profound moment, but as a series of moments of confusion and clarity. Moments of clarity were often depressing moments, where Bill realized how dramatically his life had changed because of the stroke. Whereas many stroke survivors find that they become stuck in ruminations about the devastating nature of their impairment, Bill managed to successfully push through his initial negativity to imagine ways that recovery might be possible. Much of our early conversations with Bill focused on trying to understand what motivated Bill in these initial days after waking up from the stroke.

LOSING CONTROL

"I was in the ICU for four days," Bill recalls. "Most of the time you're unconscious. You don't remember. Then you're wheeled to rehab. So, they wheeled me in and they put me in bed. The nurse came in and said, 'Your whole side is gone.' I was stuttering—I could not speak. I looked at my foot and I tried to wiggle the toe. Nothing. Tried to move my arm. Nothing. You're going, 'What the hell is this? Why can't I move?'"

"Interns will come in and say, 'What is your name?' And, of course, when you have aphasia, you can't answer. Then someone else comes in: 'Do you know where you are?' These people keep coming in and asking me questions; there are tons of people coming in. I don't know if I'm exaggerating this or not," Bill interrupts himself, "but that's what it felt like."

"People came to visit me and I didn't recognize anyone. I recognized my mom and my sister. I remember trying to tell my mom, 'Send these people away. I don't want to see anyone.'" Bill pauses, shaking his head as if to clear residual frustration. "So, you feel like you're disabled," he continues. "You don't want to talk to anyone and you're miserable."

"In one week, I dropped 35 pounds. The muscle, all the muscle in my right side is gone and so it's just skin hanging on my arm. Just bone and skin," Bill emphasizes, pinching at his right biceps. "And so, you can't get up. If you need to go to the bathroom you have to ask the nurse and she helps you get into a wheelchair."

Bill pauses for a moment, frowning slightly. "But I do remember one funny story," he blurts out, his face brightening. "The nurse in the morning would come in my room. She'd push me over, take the sheet; come on the other side, push me over, take the sheet; push me up, take the sheet off. She makes the bed while I'm in bed."

"So, she comes in and she pushes me over, and I get a whiff of this BO.[1] And I'm going, 'Oh, my God, there's nothing worse than BO.' I'm holding my breath and thinking, *Wow, this nurse needs to take a bath. Should I tell her? Because I can't even speak.* What happened was, she had moved my arm. I hadn't even realized; it was my BO!" Bill grins, transforming the dehumanizing experience of being unable to address his own hygiene into something that he can now laugh about.

"Finally, on the fourth day, they gave me a shower," he continues. "They wheeled me in and then sat me on a bench and squirted me down. I was like in prison, you know?" Bill searches our faces, checking to see if we've properly imagined the horror of losing control of one's bodily autonomy. "But, what was so frustrating is you cannot speak," he emphasizes. "They will ask you a question you cannot answer, and then they just go on doing what they have to do. Then entered my guardian angel, Susan."

***

"Do you remember a specific moment where Bill was really struggling?" Sarah presses Susan for more details.

"He was a little depressed about his stroke status," Susan remembers. "He had a bad stroke. I know—I was there. There are different levels of degrees when people have a stroke. Some have such a bad stroke it may kill them. Some people have a stroke where they're unable to utilize maybe just one part of their body or multiple parts, their limbs and things. He couldn't move one whole side of his body, and he had a kind of a droop to his lip at first."

"In the beginning, he was a very sad person. Understandably. In the beginning with Bill, I had to completely lift him with the Hoyer lift.[2] Believe it or not, he was not the man he is today. He could not walk or anything. He had to be bathed on a gurney. This made him sad, but I used to tell him, 'Bill, well, it's up to you. It's all in the mind. You can either be depressed or go ahead and work as hard as you can to overcome this. This is not an overnight thing.' When I showed him his face in the mirror, he criticized himself and said, 'God, look at me.'"

TALKING 'BOUT THE MAN IN THE MIRROR

"After introductions, she asked me, 'Would you like to see your face?'" Bill remembers, recounting his first meeting with Susan. "And I said, 'Not really.' And she says, 'You've got to see it, because you've got to do something about it.'"

---

1. An abbreviation for "body odor"

2. Hoyer lifts are used for transfers when a person requires 90% to 100% assistance to get into and out of bed. A pad fits under the person's body in the bed and connects with chains to the Hoyer lift frame. A hydraulic pump is used to lift the person off the bed surface. http://www.free-foundation.org/hoyer-lifts

"So, she brings a mirror and my whole face was distorted. UGH! Double UGH! I was ready for my performance of Quasimodo. The right side of my face had collapsed. My right eye was over an inch lower than my left eye, my mouth was almost vertical, and I just slobbered. It was not a pretty sight. Not that it's pretty now," Bill chuckles with a hint of humor, "but it wasn't pretty then. I started to cry. And lovely Susan cried with me."

***

"This was a little demeaning for him—looking like this," Susan acknowledges, "But I said, 'Bill, it's only temporary. It's up to you.' I kept telling him, 'It's up to you to recover from this. Look at that face and smile. That's you *now*; that's not going to be you later when you get better. The best thing to do is train your mind and learn how to overcome the worst by concentrating on other things like getting better, going to therapies.'"

***

"After five minutes of wallowing in self-pity, right then I knew I had to do something about my situation. 'What do I do?' I ask Susan. She rolls up a wash rag and tells me to rub it against my face to stimulate the muscles. So, with my good hand, I started doing it to help those muscles move. I did this continually until my face was sore, but I wouldn't stop. Eventually, after three days, my face was somewhat normal. There was a little sag in both my eye and my mouth, but at least I was presentable. I was determined to quit bitching about my situation and do something

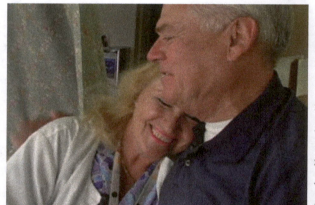

Nursing Assistant Susan Martinez and Bill

about it. Bring on the therapy! I must become independent again. I just knew I would get better; how *much* better was the big question."

THE RECOVERY BEGINS

Like most stroke survivors, Bill's recovery protocol involved several weeks of in-patient rehabilitation. Physical therapists worked on Bill's ability to balance and walk, fitting his paralyzed right foot with an AFO (Ankle Foot Orthosis) to correct its position and stabilize his weakened muscles. Occupational therapists worked with Bill's hands and arms, helping him to recover basic daily living skills like (un)dressing, (un)buttoning, and (un)zipping. Susan described how proud she was of Bill's commitment to follow through on every task assigned by his team of therapists. "He was handling it well mentally and that's what helped him get better physically," she emphasized. "That meant everything." Yet, Susan's comment downplays the vital role that she played in the early days of Bill's recovery.

THAT'S AMORE

"Well, I'm kind of the clown of the rehab," Susan laughs lightly, beaming her familiar smile. "I'm always telling jokes. I would come in and tell Bill a joke. At first, he wasn't laughing at all. I'd sit and I would say, 'Did you hear my joke?' Later, he started to laugh. Then, he started to say, 'Tell me a joke or something.' 'Yes, ah, good,' I thought, *I'm getting through to him now*."

"Then, I'd come in singing and he'd sing with me if he knew it. There's that song *Cara Mia* by Jay and the Americans. I'd come in …" Susan musters her best impression of a 1960s crooner: "Caaara Miaaaaa!" She pauses, adding, "Bill would correct me on some of the wrong words."

"He has a memory like a steel trap," Sarah quips.

"I made up a song and I sang this song to him. It's a funny song," Susan hesitates. "Shall I sing it to you?"

"Yes, I'd love to hear it!" Patricia encourages.

"You know the song by Willie Nelson, *On the Road Again*? This is my made-up song; they use it at music therapy at Scripps today still. It goes like this:

> On the commode again.
> I just can't wait to get on the commode again.
> Maalox, Mylanta, and Milk of Magnesia are my friends.
> I can't wait to get on the commode again.
> We're the best of friends, when the nurse comes with the suppository my way.
> We're the best of friends, when the nurse gives me an enema as I lay.
> On the commode again,
> I just can't wait to get on in the commode again.
> I began to think that constipation would never end.
> I can't wait to get on the commode again.

Song contributed by Susan Martinez. Copyright © Kendall Hunt Publishing Company.

We laugh together as Susan giggles, "I don't know what Willie Nelson would do if he knew what I did to his song."

After taking a moment to compose herself, Susan continues with her account of Bill's time in the hospital. "Every day I would walk in and I would just sing." She takes a deep breath and warbles the familiar opening line of Dean Martin's classic tune, "When the moon hits the sky like a big pizza pie …"

"It was just to get him smiling," she clarifies. "Eventually, he did smile and, eventually, he did converse more and more and more. He started singing it with me, eventually. It's not the only song I would walk in and sing, but it was mainly that one all the time."

"Why that song? Why *That's Amore*?" Sarah asks.

"It's just funny," Susan replies. "I can't explain why I picked that, it's just something that called his attention. When I walked in, he knew it was me."

"Day-by-day, I used to tell him, 'You can do this Bill, you can do this.' I fed him positive info all the time. Whether he could do it or not, I still made him think that he could. He got to the point where he could stand on one leg and I could help him stand up and sit on the chair, and stand up and pivot and sit on the chair. He was very happy about his improving condition. I think when he saw that he was getting better and better and better, and his therapies were helping as well, he saw that it was not a useless case."

PRO BONO THERAPY

There were many people who played a role in Bill's days, weeks, and months after waking up from his stroke. One of them was Phil Lancaster, a friend of Bill's for over 40 years who used to play paddleball with him. Phil also happened to be a physical therapist at Sharp, the hospital where Bill was originally admitted.

Since Phil was now retired, we arranged to meet him at his home for the interview. As we entered the front door of his quaint Kensington bungalow, Phil invited us to sit with him in his living room. We scooted around the bicycle parked in his entry way and sat on his comfy couch. When we asked Phil what he remembered about the day he found out his friend had been admitted to the hospital after a stroke, Phil described the shock he felt when he saw Bill's name on the hospital paperwork.

"I came to work on a Saturday morning, and I'm looking at the charts, and one of my patients is a Bill Torres," Phil remembers. "I went, 'No, it couldn't be.' I went in to look and he was asleep facing the other way. I didn't know who it was yet. I left, and I saw another patient and came back. I walked in and I was just shocked. I just went, 'Wow. Bill, what are you doing here?'"

Phil brought Bill a paper and crossword puzzle each morning and came in an hour early each day to provide extra rehab. His philosophy toward therapy was much more aggressive than that of some of his peers, particularly because he knew Bill well and guessed that he would respond well to an accelerated regimen. After a few weeks, Phil decided to push Bill beyond his comfort zone.

"I said, 'We are going to walk now,'" Phil recalls. "He looked at me and I said, 'Come on, we're walking. That's it. You're just going to have to do it.' I told him, 'OK, we're going to work on getting up off the floor.'

He said, 'What for?'

'Because you're going to fall.'

Bill said, 'No, I'm not.'

'Yes, you will.'"

"I don't know a single patient with a stroke that doesn't have a fall," Phil adds, explaining that teaching a patient how to get up after they fall is an especially important part of rehab. Even though Bill's recovery was impressively swift, he still fell one day while climbing the stairs of his mother's porch. Of course, as Phil told us with a laugh, Bill claims that he never fell; he "slid."

***

Bill's account of working with Phil is predictably much more dramatic, taking on the qualities of a Hollywood success story:

"Phil's the one who was wheeling me down the hallway on my wheelchair and I said, 'Phil, when am I going to get out of this wheelchair?'

He stopped, he put the brakes on my wheelchair, and he says, 'Just a minute.' He walked in the rehab room, came out with a cane, and he says, 'Today.'

"I panicked. I was going, 'I can't walk by myself or even with a cane.' It scared the hell out of me because I depended on that wheelchair for just about everything.

He says, 'Come on.'

Interview contributed by Philip G. Lancaster. Copyright © Kendall Hunt Publishing Company.

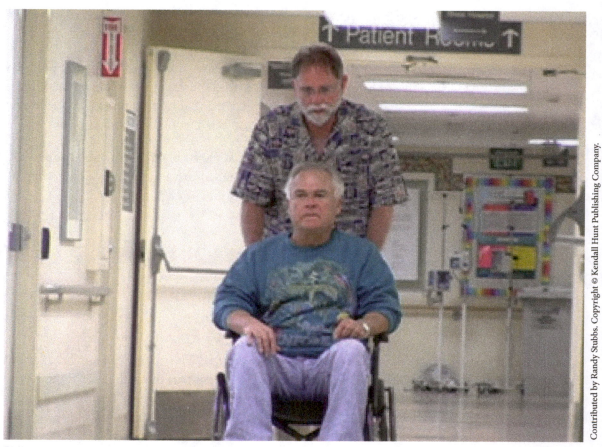

Phil Lancaster pushing Bill in a wheelchair

He got me up, and I left the wheelchair."

Both Phil and Bill describe this moment—the day Bill stood up—as an "ah-ha" moment that opened up a lot of possibilities for recovery. That turning point moment led to others, including Phil getting Bill on a stationary bike, tying Bill's "bad" foot to the pedal, and challenging him to pedal for thirty minutes. Bill tells us, "I never missed one minute of therapy—not one minute."

CLOSING REFLECTIONS

When do you wake up from stroke? Is it when you realize you can't move one whole side of your body? Is it when you look in the mirror and see a face you don't recognize? Is it when you try to tell someone something and find that you can't express yourself? Waking from stroke is a continuous process; the survivor is awakened from one moment to the next as they come to new realizations about their transformed body and experience new emotions about their transformed reality. Just as every stroke is different, so, too, is a person's response to and awareness of what is happening to them.

For Bill, waking up from his stroke was both a relief and a devastation. Bill was relieved that he didn't die and that his mom would not face the death of a second child. But once the reality of what he would face in the long road to recovering from stroke hit him, Bill, like most stroke survivors, faced intense depression when he realized how far he must travel to speak, to walk, to do all the things he had taken for granted. But unlike many stroke survivors who want to get lost in TV, in sleep, or in anything that will take their minds away from the devastation they feel, Bill took action with support and assistance from health care providers like Susan and friends like Phil.

Bill spent one month in the hospital and then three months being driven to and from rehab three times a week. That one month in the hospital was vital for his survivorship. Nurses like Susan and physical therapists like Phil played a critical role, not only in assisting his physical recovery but also in inspiring him mentally to want to improve in the days and weeks after his stroke. Susan offered a mindset of success and positivity, saying, "You can do this Bill, you can do this," or "That's you now. That's not going to be you later when you get better." Her approach was playful and engaging; singing songs, telling jokes, and having her own entrance song with "That's Amore." She pushed through the mental barriers that Bill might have formed to engage him and create a powerful relationship that they both still remember affectionately over 15 years later. Phil, as both Bill's long-term friend and physical therapist, offered Bill what other therapists might not have been able to offer—an intimate understanding of Bill's identity and an innately trusting relationship.

Yet the foundations for Bill's recovery were forged long before his hospital stay. In the following chapter, we return to an exploration of earlier phases of Bill's life, seeking to understand how Bill developed the restless desire for self-improvement that would form the core of his post-stroke recovery efforts.

CHAPTER 4

"So, Bill, how's the clean-shaven face? Are you sticking with that?" Patricia asks as breakfast arrives: Mediterranean omelets loaded with black olives, tomatoes, feta cheese, and basil. We've settled into our booth at Lake Murray Café. Bill has scraped away the white stubble he'd sported during our last visit, revealing a square jaw and swarthy skin—surprisingly smooth for a man in his 80s.

"Oh, yeah, I stopped with the beard a long time ago," Bill replies with a wave of his hand.

"Did you like the beard or …" Patricia probes.

"Oh, it was something different," Bill shrugs. "You know, I get bored with my life."

Bill's eyes turn uncharacteristically serious, set in the folds of his laugh lines. "I'm kind of a lost soul. I'm always searching for something different. Even though I can feed the birds ten years without missing any days, I like a little adventure, a little change. I'm tired of teaching here, I'll go teach someplace else. When I had my stroke, I was going to teach in Japan. I'm always searching for something."

"When we ended our interview last time, you were telling us about the time that you were teaching in a special program. Is that right?" Patricia asks.

"A special program?"

"For the oil company," Sarah clarifies.

"That wasn't a special program," Bill says, "I was just teaching down in South America."

***

It was 1965. Bill had spent the last three years teaching 5th and 6th grade at Emerson Elementary School in San Diego, but now he was feeling restless. While flipping through a copy of *Instructor Magazine*, a photo of a tropical paradise caught his eye. "Teach in Venezuela!" the caption commanded; it was an advertisement for a program organized by Standard Oil. Bill took the chance and applied. He soon found himself teaching a class of six 7th and 8th graders near the company's massive oil refinery in the city of Amuay.

A fishing port nestled in the curve of a natural bay, Amuay sits on the beach-rich Paraguana Peninsula three hours from Venezuela's capital, Caracas. Amuay, as one of the biggest towns on the peninsula, is named Judibana, which means "strong winds" in the local tongue. Twenty-five-mile-per-hour gusts stream steadily from the ocean, mitigating the sultry heat. Standard Oil had planted palm trees to transform the desert into an oasis for its employees. They put Bill up in a large, U-shaped house with no less than 16 doors opening onto its courtyard; rent was US$25 per month. At the bayside tennis courts, the locals rig cloth sheets to shield their play from the wind. Bill learned how to hit the ball at just the right angle so that it would blow back onto the court, boomerang style. By 1967, however, Bill found himself on a boomerang path back to his old life in the United States.

***

"Two years was enough," Bill says.

"What happened from there to get you back to the U.S.?" Patricia asks.

"I was 30-years-old, right? What goes through a young man's mind at 30-years-old?"

"Looking for a partner—a life partner," Patricia nods.

"Right. There wasn't … you couldn't date the girls at …" Bill pauses, then settles into the cushioned diner booth. "I'll tell you one story …"

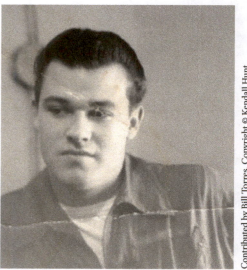

Bill at age 31, 1966

JOSEFINA

"I fly into Caracas—that's the largest city in Venezuela. They have this nice hotel, the Tequendama Hotel. Women didn't go to bars there, or if they did go, they went with their parents. I was disappointed; I went bar hopping looking for a woman. I came back to the hotel. I'd just gotten into bed, and my phone rings.

'Mr. Torres?'

'Yes?'

'Is the music bothering you?'

'No, but what music?'

'Well, there's a big wedding down here and they're getting loud. I'm just checking to see if it's okay. We can move you.'

'No, that's alright. Who got married?'

'Well, oddly enough, someone named Torres.'

I hung up. I put my suit back on, got a drink at the bar, and walked into the reception. I said, 'My name is Torres.' I showed them my ID, and they let me right in.

I saw this young, beautiful woman sitting there with her sister and mom and dad, and I went over and asked her to dance. Her name was Josefina Torres. She didn't speak one word of English. At that time, my Spanish was a little better than what it is now, and I said, 'I'd like to come back to Caracas and take you out.'

She said, 'Well, let me ask my mother and father.'

We go back and sit and they liked me, and they said, 'Well sure, yes.'

The next week, I was 180 miles from Caracas in Amuay. I took a two hour flight back to the capital and rented a car—a little Renault. I found their house, a big, beautiful home. I go up there and knock on the door and she's ready. But who's coming along with her? Her grandmother and her sister.

So, we have dinner. We laugh and they stumble through my Spanish. Her sister could speak English fluently, which was good. I said, 'How about if I come in a couple of weeks and we'll go out again?' And she goes, 'OK.' I take them home. It was a good night.

A couple of weeks later I fly back in. I go up there and this time it's just her sister. She says, 'I can bring my boyfriend with me.' I had to treat her boyfriend, because I'm a rich American.

I said, 'Are we ever going to be alone?'

I come back in a couple of weeks. I go in their house, and there are balloons all over—helium balloons on the ceiling. I'm going, 'What's happening?'

She says, 'Well, there's going to be a party later.'

I said, 'wonderful.'

So, we go out to dinner—just the two of us. As the night wore on, she kept getting sadder and sadder.

'Are you okay?' I ask.

'Yes, I'm okay.' And I'm thinking, *What the hell is going on here?*

'Do you want to go home?'

'Yes.' And I'm wondering, *What the hell did I do? Bad breath? Body odor?*

We go home. I go up with her and open the door, and the whole family is there screaming, 'Surprise! Yay!' Then, complete silence.

I said, 'What's happening?'

Her sister comes over and she asks, 'Bill, you didn't give her an engagement ring? This is an engagement party.'

I said, 'I'm sorry, I didn't know. I'm from the United States. I don't know your way of life. I'm very sorry if I hurt anyone.'

'All right, you'd better just leave.'

I left. There must have been a hundred and fifty people there, and I'm gone. That's why I came back to the United States."

***

We laugh together as Bill delivers the punchline; so many of his stories have the larger-than-life quality of a movie plot. "When you came back, what happened?" Patricia prompts. "You didn't go back to teaching at your old school, did you?

"Yes, I did. For six months, I just fooled around. I had a ton of money because I didn't spend much when I was living in Amuay. But, in the summer of '66, between the two years I was teaching in Venezuela, I had come back to visit San Diego and met a young lady …"

***

As an employee of Standard Oil, Bill was permitted to hitch a ride on any of the many oil tankers that docked in Amuay's busy port, as long as he asked the ship's owner for permission. So, Bill ended up telegraphing the Greek shipping magnate, Aristotle Onassis—paramour to the famed opera singer, Maria Callas, future husband to the widowed Jackie Kennedy, and one of the richest men of the time period. Armed with a return telegraph from Onassis himself, and with his one-dollar fare, Bill secured passage aboard the *Olympic Splendor*, the day before it set out for San Francisco. The ship was as grimy and inelegantly industrial as any tanker, but Bill took up residence in Onassis's opulent, chandelier-festooned suite. The crew were convinced that he must be quite wealthy.

Bill spent much of the 12-day trip topside, wearing shorts and no shirt. He cultivated a thick, dark beard and a deep tan. When the ship passed through the Panama Canal, the American pilots guiding them through the locks mistook Bill for some South American traveler. Bill pointed at the locomotive-like contraption that was guiding the tanker through the canal with cables and winches. "What's that name?" he mimicked in halting English.

"That … is … called … a … mule," one pilot replied, exaggerating each word.

"Yes, a mule," the other emphasized, pantomiming a donkey. "Hee haw, hee haw."

The ship's captain began cracking up, spoiling Bill's ruse. "I'm just pulling your leg—I'm American," Bill admitted.

The pilots laughed good naturedly, pointing to their colleague across the deck. "Get him next!"

The trip took the long 12 days because it was slowed by a storm off the coast of Mexico. When Bill finally hopped a flight home from San Francisco to San Diego, all he wanted was a burger and fries from Jack-in-the-Box. When an old friend tracked him down and told him he had a girl he wanted him to meet, Bill was decidedly less than enthusiastic. He was, after all, planning to return to Venezuela. He came out for a drink at the Hilton lobby bar and met the young woman, but didn't think much of the encounter.

Several weeks later, Bill found himself back on a flight to San Francisco on his way to renew his visa. He'd had a bit too much to drink the night before, so he had slept too late to catch any of the earlier flights to San Francisco. He ended up on the last flight of the day, slumped in one of the first-row seats with dark glasses hiding his bleary eyes. He had only just fallen asleep when he heard someone call his name, and felt someone tug his glasses from the bridge of his nose. He blinked into the lovely face of the flight attendant—the same woman he'd met in the Hilton lobby.

***

"After I returned to Venezuela, she was writing me all the time," Bill tells us. "I was falling in love with her letters because I didn't have anyone to fall in love with in Venezuela. Everything seemed so important. We didn't have Internet or anything." Bill pauses and grins roguishly at Sarah. "You know what a letter is?"

"Yes, she does!" Patricia laughs.

"Anyway, I started going with her and eventually married her," Bill continues.

"What was her name?" Patricia asks.

"Ursula," Bill replies. "I married her at the end of '67, October. I had a wonderful 2 years, 4 months, 12 days, 9 hours, 25 minutes and 2 seconds of marriage. Then, I got divorced."

Sarah raises her eyebrows and glances over at Patricia. "I think we're about to hear another one of Bill's stories."

URSULA

Ursula was from Germany. She had grown up in a well-appointed flat above her parents' various businesses—a luggage shop, a barber shop, a beauty salon, and a perfume shop. When the bombs of World War II destroyed their home and livelihood, the family fled Europe for the United States to live with cousins in Milwaukee, Wisconsin.

Once in America, Ursula's father began an affair. He brought his paramour home to have dinner with his wife, claiming that she was new to town and in need of friends. Eventually, Ursula's mother began to notice that her husband was making a habit of returning at two or three o'clock in the morning after driving to their guest home, alleging car trouble or some other excuse. She and 17-year-old Ursula packed up their belongings and took the train to San Diego.

Mother and daughter took jobs as seamstresses at May Company, a fashionable Los Angeles-based department store chain founded in the 1920s. Over the next few years, Ursula's father pleaded for them to return: "Come back to Milwaukee. Come join me in Cologne." Each time, they went. Each time, they found that he was still unfaithful. He blamed his infidelities on the influence of American culture: "You know, it's the United States. It's corrupted my mind. They don't have any morality here, and I'm falling into it."

Bill met Ursula when she was 24 and working as a flight attendant for Pacific Southwest (PSA), America's first discount airline headquartered in San Diego. On visits to Ursula's home, his future mother-in-law doted on him in her heavy German accent: "Did you eat? Oh, you're a bachelor— your shirt is missing a button! Let me button that for you. Take your shirt off, let me fix that." Her solicitousness did the trick; Bill proposed to her daughter soon after his teaching gig in Venezuela dried up. While the young couple was not destined for a lastingly happy marriage, their first few months as newlyweds included some memorable adventures—including the vacation of a lifetime.

***

It all began with a bag of tea.

Ursula was working a commuter route, flying three times a day between San Diego, Los Angeles, and San Francisco. She befriended one of the regulars on her 8 a.m. flight—a woman who preferred tea as the source of her morning caffeine. At the time, Pacific Southwest Airlines didn't serve anything but coffee to its patrons, so Ursula took to buying her own tea and bringing a sachet for her friend.

One evening, Ursula came home from work. "Have you ever been to Acapulco?" she asked her young husband, naming Mexico's booming beachside resort town.

"Yes," Bill replied.

"Well, I haven't."

"We'll go there sometime," Bill responded, trying to placate his young wife.

"Yes, we *can* go there," Ursula said, "There's this lady on the plane who I serve tea to. She has a hotel down in Acapulco and she asked me if we'd like to come down there as her guests. When could we go?"

Bill suggested that they could make the trip over Easter Break, when he'd be off from school. After they'd made the arrangements with the lady from the plane, however, he began to worry. Easter Break would be Semana Santa,[1] a popular time for local Mexican tourists to visit Acapulco. Feeling guilty for taking rooms for free during a prime time, he called the lady and offered to book his own lodgings elsewhere. "Bill, this is a special hotel," she told him, "I don't want you to worry about a thing."

Ursula and Bill paid US$6 to take a PSA flight down to Mexico. When they disembarked, however, Bill immediately lowered his expectations for their vacation. *They haven't even sent a car to pick us up from the airport*, he thought as they claimed their baggage and hailed a cab. *This must be a cheap hotel.* He and Ursula settled into the back of a rather beat-up looking taxi. "Acapulco Towers, please," he instructed the driver. "Si, señor!" the cabbie replied enthusiastically. Bill turned to his wife. "Ursula, this guy's eyes just lit up when I mentioned the name of our hotel," he whispered. Bill had stayed in Acapulco several times before, including at the Ritz and at the Hilton, but he'd never heard of this place. He decided to gather some intel. "Señor," he called to the driver, "How is that hotel?"

"Mejor, mejor!" the man enthused, "You're going to fall in love with it." He turned up a road that wended its way over and around the hills surrounding Acapulco, climbing upward until the three

1. "Celebrated in basically every Spanish-speaking country, la Semana Santa (*Holy Week*) is the week leading up to Easter, the highest of Catholic holy days. It's full of prayers and masses in preparation for Easter Sunday. It is very typical to see many procesiones, or *religious processions* take place throughout cities in Latin America" (para. 5). https://www.spanishdict.com/guide/a-year-of-celebrations-in-spanish-speaking-countries

impressive buildings comprising Acapulco Towers came into view. Perched on a ridge, the hotel's numerous verandas offered expansive views of the city below and the glistening waves of the Pacific. The grounds looked impeccably maintained; lush gardens filled with flowering hibiscus offered invitingly shady places to sit and sip a margarita. Bill and Ursula emerged from their cab and stood in stunned silence as the manager rushed up to greet them, rattling on in Spanish. "I'm sorry," he said, switching to English once he realized that they were Americans, "Our limousine broke down and we could not send it. We will be sure to make it up to you."

The manager guided Bill and Ursula to their room—a two-bedroom suite with a balcony and a well-appointed kitchen stocked with beer, whiskey, and wine. "We didn't know what you like to drink, so we included everything," the manager shrugged apologetically, just as the lady from the plane arrived with two banana daiquiris in hand. "Ursula, this is the best hotel," Bill told his wife once the manager and their host had gone. "There are even real painting on the walls!"

As dinner time approached, Bill and Ursula made their way to the bar in search of food. "What's your name?" Bill asked the sole bartender as he fixed their margaritas.

"They call me 'Cookie,' since I'm the cook," the man responded.

"Where is everyone, Cookie?" Bill asked, gesturing to the empty bar area and the vacant veranda.

"You are the only guests, Mr. Torres."

"Oh," Bill replied, momentarily speechless. "Well, we'd like to have dinner. Are there any menus?"

"Order whatever you'd like to eat. I'll make it," Cookie said, guiding them to a seat on the hibiscus-festooned veranda.

"Well my wife likes hippopotamus and I like rhino," Bill joked.

"We don't have *that*," Cookie laughed. "Anything else?"

They made do with lobster tails, beans and rice, and fresh tortillas, inviting Cookie to sit with them as they ordered another round of margaritas. "Tell us about this place, Cookie," they encouraged.

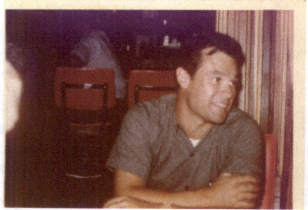

Bill in his 30s

"A lot of famous people come here. Are you famous?"

"No, no. I'm a schoolteacher and she's a flight attendant."

"You're rich?" Cookie tried.

"No, no. I'm a school teacher!" Bill repeated, laughing.

"Well, a lot of famous people come here. You'll see—tomorrow," Cookie promised.

The next day, Bill and Ursula took the repaired limousine into town to go shopping. They laughed at how the limo followed behind them as they strolled from store to store, making them feel like Hollywood movie stars. When they returned to Acapulco Towers for the happy hour, they were no longer the only guests drinking banana daiquiris on the veranda. Bill glanced around at the posh clientele, slurping his tropical cocktail through a colorful straw. He paused mid-sip as a strikingly familiar figure strode passed their table.

"Ursula," he whispered, nodding toward the man surreptitiously. "Is that … Frank Sinatra?"

"I think it is!" Ursula gasped, eyes widening above her daiquiri's whipped cream.

"Cookie," Bill called, beckoning to the bartender. "See those people over there?"

"Oh, yeah. Mr. Sinatra. He comes here all the time."

"Buy him a drink on me." Bill and Ursula watched with glee as Cookie brought a drink to Sinatra and his companion, Steve Lawrence.[2]

"Thank you, Mr. Torres!" Sinatra waved, acknowledging the gesture.

"No, it's just Bill, Mr. Sinatra!"

"Well, it's just Frank here," Sinatra replied, sending a drink to them in return.

By the end of their week-long stay, it became pretty clear that the lady from the plane was not just any random tea lover. She was, in fact, "Mrs. M.," the heiress for a major condiment company. And, as is typical of an uber rich person, Mrs. M. asked Bill to complete a seemingly impossible favor on the way back to San Diego. She had a piece of pottery that she wanted Bill and Ursula to carry back with them to the United States. Yet, as Bill discovered when he picked the piece up from the hotel

2. Steve Lawrence is a 1960s-era singer and actor, best known for duo "Steve and Eydie" with his late wife Eydie Gormé. "They accompanied Sinatra on his last world tour. They partied with him in Las Vegas. They stayed with Frank and Barbara Sinatra at their Rancho Mirage compound. In fact, Lawrence is one of the few singers legally entitled to use Sinatra's arrangements today" (Fessier, 2016, para 1).

manager, this wasn't the kind of bowl that you can buy from Pier One. It was a beautiful example of pre-Columbian pottery—a museum-worthy artifact that would certainly be illegal to transport across national borders.

Bill felt quite indebted to Mrs. M., so he racked his brain for a plan to fulfill her request. He remembered an old joke about a thief who carried a wheelbarrow filled with straw out of town each day. The town's guard always stopped and inspected the contents of the thief's wheelbarrow, but never discovered anything amiss. One day, the guard implored the thief, "Please, I know that you are stealing something, but I can't figure out what it is! Just tell me your secret—I won't turn you in."

"Well," the thief replied with a saucy grin, "I've been stealing wheelbarrows."

Who knew that an old joke would contain the directions for successful international smuggling? Bill and Ursula carefully filled the fragile bowl with several wrapped parcels. As anticipated, the customs agents scrutinized the packages without giving the vessel a second glance. Bill, Ursula, and Mrs. M.'s pre-Columbian pottery made it home to San Diego without incident.

⁎

While Bill's marriage to Ursula began with the kind of fairytale feel of an Acapulco getaway, the young couple soon ran into problems. When they'd married, Bill had no idea that Ursula's parents' marital drama had so heavily damaged Ursula's capacity for trust. The details of her family history only emerged when he insisted that they see a psychologist after Ursula repeatedly accused him of cheating. Her suspicions deepened when Bill enrolled in law school; he spent his evenings away from Ursula, studying at the library late into the night. Eventually, Ursula turned to alcohol to dull the ache of her neuroses. As her alcoholism worsened, Bill was reminded of his father's own battle with addiction. It was time to leave.

⁎

"One day I just said, 'Goodbye.'" Bill tells us. "I walked out of the house, a beautiful home up at Mission Hills. I moved in with her mother."

"With Ursula's mother?" Patricia asks, incredulous.

"Yes, her mother had a room," Bill laughs. "Her mother realized that her daughter was going crazy. I lived with her for about three months. I told Ursula, 'You can have everything. The only thing I want is out.'"

FALLING IN LOVE WITH THE PROCESS: CULTIVATING RESILIENCE IN HEALTH CRISES

I went back to my house and the only thing left was an iron skillet. She took all of my books—I had hundreds. She didn't read. I asked her, 'Why did you take all my books?' She said, 'Why, I have shelves in here and they need books.'

Anyway, I guess it was seven to eight years later that she passed away. She was only 35, 36. Beautiful. Then the mother died of a broken heart; she died a couple of weeks after the funeral." Bill pauses briefly, giving us the space of a few seconds to wonder at how such painful events could be stated so matter-of-factly. "Kids aren't supposed to die before their parents," he continues. "My sister died when she was like 57, 58-years-old."

"Really? Patricia asks. What did she die of?"

"We don't know."

"You don't know?" Patricia responds, intrigued.

"Come on, Bill, you can't leave us in suspense," Sarah pushes. "What happened?"

GLORIA

Bill's youngest sister, Joanne, moved with her husband to Leadville, Colorado, where he worked mining molybdenum for the U.S. steel industry. The couple had two young children, and Bill's oldest sister, Gloria, moved to Colorado to care for them. Gloria found her own husband there, and the two sisters and their families lived in Leadville for 17 years—until Gloria began exhibiting some disturbing symptoms. The local hospital diagnosed her with schizophrenia, but Bill was convinced that something else had happened to Gloria. He urged Joanne, "Put her on a plane, bring her down to San Diego, get her here in the hospital."

Gloria got off the plane in a daze. She could barely talk, one eye was drooping, and one arm had curled itself up toward her chest. San Diegan doctors confirmed that Gloria had had a stroke. Bill settled his sister in a house across the street from his mother's mobile home. She never quite regained her mobility or her ability to speak

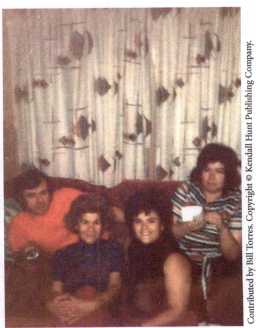

Contributed by Bill Torres. Copyright © Kendall Hunt Publishing Company.

Left to right: Bill, Bill's mom (Babe), and sisters, Joanne and Gloria, 1963 fluently. When Gloria got sick a few years later and her mother could not care for her, they moved her into a rest home.

***

"I remember going down to see her," Bill says. "The staff was going to move her back to the hospital, give her some more tests. They said, 'You can pick her up tomorrow morning.' I went over to my mother's house. We were getting ready to go to the hospital to pick Gloria up when the phone rang:

'Your sister passed away last night.'

'Of what?'

'We don't know, they're doing an autopsy.'

I said, 'Mom, Gloria passed. They want to do an autopsy.'

She said, 'No, bring her home. I don't want them cutting her up.'"

"That death must have been hard on your mom," Patricia suggests.

"That devastated my mom," Bill agrees. "And that's why I said to you that I couldn't die. When I was in the middle of having a stroke, I'd come to and think, *Am I going to die this time? I can't die. My mother is still alive.* I just had a will to live. Afterward, I felt like that was the only reason why I lived—because I knew that if I died, my mother would die."

CLOSING REFLECTIONS

What is Bill "always searching" for? Stories like Bill's account of applying to teach in Venezuela suggest an indefatigable desire for adventure. Unable to sit still, Bill is a man of constant—often impulsive—action. This character trait served Bill well during his recovery from stroke. Never content with the status quo, Bill channeled his restlessness into seeking creative ways to address and minimize his physical impairments.

Yet Bill's "lost soul" yearns for something deeper and more fundamental than new scenery. He is also searching for connection. Bill is the kind of person who will return to the duck pond every morning for ten years, because he knows that Philip the Goose will be waiting for a bite of birdseed. He is the kind of person who will fly to another city (three times) to take a woman he's just met out on a date. He is the kind of person who, in the midst of having a stroke, thinks first about how his death will impact the people he loves. As with so many of the things in his life, Bill's recovery and subsequent advocacy work are motivated by his sense of connection with, and obligation to, others. In some ways, Bill's emotional experience of going through stroke strengthened his sense of connection even further. In the next chapter, we delve deeper into the ways Bill's experience of stroke threatened his identity, producing difficult emotional hurdles.

REFERENCE

Fessier, B. (2016, February 9). Singer Steve Lawrence remembers mentor Frank Sinatra. *The Desert Sun*. Retrieved from https://www.desertsun.com/story/life/entertainment/music/2016/02/08/singer-steve-lawrence-remembers-mentor-frank-sinatra/79905916/

CHAPTER 5

"You ready for some stuff?" Bill asks, "It's all color-coded. Don't mind me." Sarah laughs as Bill passes out several stacks of paper, neatly bundled with colorful paperclips. They are a treasure trove of stories, each carefully titled and typed in baby blue, 16-point Calibri.

"This is awesome," Sarah enthuses.

"I'll give you each copies. I made copies for all three of us."

"These are great. Excellent, Bill! Boy, he does his homework, doesn't he?" Patricia says.

"He is a great student."

"Don't go away," Bill says, continuing to pass out packets. "This one's titled 'Tap Dancing.' This is one that broke my heart. This is 'Delray.' I don't know how to—sometimes I don't use a subjunctive, I do whatever sounds better. I know that you're going to change them because you're women."

"What?!" Sarah exclaims in mock outrage. "Because we're *intelligent*."

"Intelligent women," Bill chuckles, "They're the worst kind."

"Nooo," Sarah insists through her laughter.

"That's 'Rose,'" Bill continues. "That was a wonderful story. This one is classic. This is 'John and Marcia.' This is 'Thai Lady of the Lake.' And this one," Bill pauses, "Is 'My Stroke.'" Two blue words scream in all caps from the top of the page: 'WHY ME.'

***

That's the first thing I thought when I came out of a three-day coma and was being pushed down a long hall to rehab ... WHY ME? WHY ME? Each morning when you wake you're hoping it's all a bad dream. But that fades fast when you try to move your hand, arm, or foot. Nothing. Your mind is screaming, "Damn, damn nothing." Again, again and again "WHY ME?" Then, once the rage has subsided, you again say, "what next?"

Now I know why I have waited so long to put this in writing … when I speak about my stroke to rotary clubs, college classes, individuals, and so on, the words disappear after I've concluded with the presentation. But now the words are in front of me and my memories are flooded with hate for that time when I struggled for eight months just to move a finger. But I digress.

Every day was a new adventure; "Let's see if there is any progress." Still nothing! Three hours, and nothing. "Oh well, there's always tomorrow."

I would go back to my hospital room and scream into my pillow. I'd take ten minutes every evening and scream, "Why me? Why am I this way? What did I do wrong?" I just got all the negativity out of me, screaming louder. Then I took off the pillow before imagining what would happen tomorrow. Phil's going to come in early. He's going to bring me the *New York Times'* crossword puzzle. He's going to wheel me over and tie my foot to the bike and have me pedal for a half hour.

I was determined to quit bitching about my situation and do something about it. I made a promise to myself that if I got better, I would become an advocate for stroke survivors. More on this later.

***

"You were asking me, 'What made you this way?'" Bill says, responding to our questions about how he managed to be so remarkably resilient in the wake of his stroke. "One of the reasons why I got better was vanity. I didn't want people seeing me disabled.

When I had lunch with a friend that came to pick me up from the hospital when I was released, she thought she was doing me a favor. What I wanted, I wanted to go home and hide. I'm in a wheelchair.

So, she takes me down the fish market and I'm like, 'Oh my god. I'm going to be wheeled down in there, and I swear'—People really aren't looking at you, but you know they are."

"You feel it," Patricia nods.

"You can feel it. They had pity on me, and I hated that feeling. We went down there, we ordered fish. It was nice, but I didn't want to be there. I wanted to be home and hide under the covers."

"But your friends wouldn't let you hide?" Sarah probes.

"No, they wouldn't," Bill agrees. "You'll meet my friend, Charlie, tomorrow. He was a five-time national champion racquetball player. I was pretty good, but Charlie was in a class by himself. I was lucky to get a couple of points out of Charlie—that's how good he was. And he's brilliant; graduated USD, summa cum laude both in undergrad and grad."

"What's his area?" Sarah asks.

"Attorney. He was the top of his class. The only thing he could never control was his temper. He's loud, very intelligent, thinks outside the box all the time, but he is a good guy …."

"PEOPLE DON'T EVEN WANNA SEE YOU WHEN THEY'RE EATING": CHARLIE

"He claims I caused his stroke," Charlie says, brown eyes sparkling with mischief behind large, wire-rimmed glasses. His voice has the resonant clarity of a radio personality, despite the fact that he is obviously quite ill. Tumors from metastatic prostate cancer have made his bones exceptionally brittle; his narrow face is pale underneath the close-cropped gray scruff of his beard and mustache. Bill gave Charlie a ride here, helping him to maneuver into a chair across from us in a seating area outside the therapists' offices at the Sharp Grossmont Hospital Outpatient Rehabilitation Center.

Charlie flashes a bright, lopsided grin, rekindling the swagger of a former racquetball champion. "We were playing racquetball the day before the stroke," he continues. "Because he was so proficient at the way he played, he never moved. By the way, I didn't mention he was slow as fuck. And so, I had great control of the ball and my specialty was called the 'tour of the court,' where I would punish my opponent. So, I was trying to break Bill of the habit of standing around. I was running him back and forth to where, later, when I finally caught up with him at the rehab center after the stroke, he was going, 'You son of a bitch!'" Charlie's roguish smile reemerges, transforming Bill's stroke into fodder for good-natured trash talking.

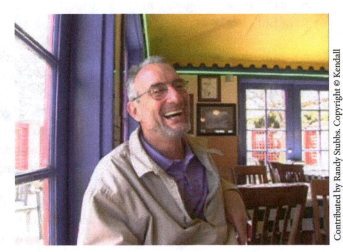

Charlie Brumfield

"We were responsible for some medical changes in the way they ran the department when I visited the hospital," Charlie smirks. "They let him go on a tour with me in the facility with the wheelchair, and I picked up speed. And when we hit the ledge, he was ready to catapult out. He couldn't move his arms. And after that, they changed the policy to have seatbelts—and we're responsible," Charlie laughs.

"So, we started going walking. And we have an old joke still to this day; we debated all the time because we'd be walking around the neighborhood for a half a mile or whatever and then I'd say, 'Let's go down this slightly declining dirt area.' And he goes, 'I can't walk on uneven ground.' And I go, 'Bullshit! Come with me and we'll go down the uneven and then you're gonna be able to walk on uneven ground. You'll try an even more arduous task,' which is my approach.

So, he insisted that the main feature of his recovery was not falling. He didn't take what I would call a risk approach, which I would have," Charlie adds, gesturing with a slender arm. "Because I'm not gonna voluntarily stay at whatever level here if I think that by doing something risky I can get to the level here." Charlie pauses, suddenly becoming self-conscious of the fact that he's been rambling. "Let's go back to the question, so I'm not freewheeling," he says.

"No, you've actually answered a lot of the questions," Sarah reassures. "I'm trying to figure out which ones we didn't get … I guess one of the things that we can't get from a lot of folks is the direct aftermath of Bill's stroke—"

"First thing that I noticed," Charlie cuts in, "is that it's so embarrassing to be helpless and to be deformed because your muscles don't even work, and your face, and you can't speak." Charlie settles into his chair and adopts a more contemplative tone. "People have that problem to begin with. Non-stroke people have it as well. That's why they've got this billion-dollar industry where people will spend to make themselves look better so that they feel they can walk out the door. But in the position of a stroke survivor, it's the extreme. Their minds work, but they feel like the elephant man. They don't wanna be seen. They don't wanna be touched.

You gotta understand that these stroke survivors were flawed human beings before. They're Americans. And they have been raised in a carnal situation where there's significant problems, which is part of the wall that goes up. The wall is a reflection of an evil principle taught by Madison Avenue. Unless you're beautiful, unless you can speak like the angels, don't talk. Be over here and please, we don't wanna see you while we're eating. You know, that type of thing. And that's the thing that you feel worst about. People don't even wanna see you when they're eating. I even start tearing up when I start thinking of that concept.

I was a drug addict. That's why I know quite a bit about the issues we're talking about. I once wondered—I had like 1,000 friends and people with money that would help me. I once thought, *Well, how would I do if I was a minority member who didn't have any support, whatsoever?* So, you know, I don't want to ever take away from Bill's achievements, but he had friends. And those friends came out to see him and made him comfortable with who he was at that time."

"Oh, I'll tell you a story," Charlie continues, the familiar smile returning. "Bill's quite the womanizer."

"We figured that out," Patricia laughs. "We got that day one."

"OK," Charlie says, "Bill comes to me and goes, 'Charles, I got the golden opportunity.' I go, 'What is it?' He says, 'I'm going around the world in my sailboat and I'm recruiting coeds from state college as my crew.' I go, 'Oh really, Bill, that's gonna go well.' So, he gathers all these girls up. They take off, and a hurricane hits him ten miles down the coast and they crash. And I go, 'Bill—karma. Karma.'"

We laugh together in the moment it takes for Charlie to turn more thoughtful. "But what he said that was like a stroke survivor," Charlie recalls, "he said, 'When I turned 50, I was invisible when I walked into a bar.' That's a derivation of the same principle we're discussing now. You know, the issue of being invisible after 50 is almost another aspect of 'they don't wanna eat around me.'

I mean, I've got the same problems. I mean, I can feel it. I suffer from that, and I gotta work on that, and I'd like to finish before the conclusion of …" Charlie pauses. "I'm getting up there. It's getting pretty tricky. That 4th colostomy bag is a little heavy."

***

"What happens when you have the stroke, those neurons are destroyed," Bill explains, seated at Patricia's oak dining room table. "Those connections are gone. Now, a lot of things that you learned as a kid are gone. You have to relearn them all. You have to learn to tie your shoes over again. So, one of the things when a boy is growing up, if you cry, what does your dad tell you? 'Hey, big boys do not cry. Be tough, be a man, be a macho marine thing.' And that's destroyed. So, I cried at anything. I would watch the *Seinfeld* episode of George screwing up. I would cry for George." Sarah smiles, imagining Bill sobbing over the canned audience laughter of a 1990s sitcom.

"Then, those connections start coming back and then you don't do that," Bill continues. "But I still haven't lost the cry. If I'm sitting all alone, I can just be watching TV, and everything strikes me. It's emotional, but I can control it now.

So, I don't judge anyone by their emotion. Especially when you have a stroke, all different emotions come out. Mean. You can get mean. Especially guys, they get very angry. And the first ones that they are angry at are their spouses."

"Really?" Patricia asks.

"Oh, yeah. Or most guys—most of the guys between 30 and 40 want to commit suicide."

"We're interviewing a younger guy—Russell—tomorrow," Sarah says.

"Russell?" Bill asks. "I didn't know you were going to talk to him …." When Bill itemized a list of who we should talk to, he did mention Russell as a young man who had a stroke, who Bill had talked to and encouraged at the hospital. But that was awhile back and he didn't know until this moment that we had set up a time to interview Russell.

"I JUST CRY SOMETIMES …. I WARN EVERYBODY": RUSSELL

"I moved to San Diego in 2008 and almost a year after I moved here—it was March 2009—I had a stroke," Russell begins. Sarah, Patricia, and Russell are waiting for their iced coffees to arrive, sitting on small stools around a tall wooden table in a trendy North Park coffee shop. Russell looks to be in his mid to late thirties, with closely cropped brown hair, a defined jawline, and the barrel-shaped chest of a former athlete. He agreed to be interviewed after Sarah e-mailed to describe our book project with Bill—one of the people who inspired Russell's post-stroke recovery.

"I got really dizzy when I was washing the dishes and then I just sat down. Then I couldn't talk," Russell continues. "I was trying to talk to my girlfriend, and she finally looked over like, 'What are you doing? Let's go.' I lifted my right hand and dropped it and I couldn't move it. She had been a lifeguard, so she had some knowledge and she kind of knew what it was, but then didn't believe it because I was young."

"How old were you?" Sarah asks.

"Twenty-nine. I was going to be 30 soon. She goes to call the ambulance and I'm like, 'Mhhhh.' I don't want to. I'm cheap," Russell adds sheepishly.

"Before you call the cops, let me get my calculator out here," Sarah says, pantomiming frantic calculations.

"Yes," Russell says. "I stood up and I was holding the chair with one hand, and we tried to walk to the car. I went to step with my right leg and just fell. We tried again, and fell again, and she's like, 'This is it, I am calling an ambulance.' And I'm like, 'No, no, no, no.' But I couldn't talk, so she goes and gets my neighbor—she got this little 90-pound woman across the hallway."

"It's like me!" Sarah laughs.

"Yes," Russell says. "They got me into my office chair and wheeled me around to the car. And then I start taking my clothes off because I know in all the movies they cut your shorts and they cut your shirt. I don't want them to cut my clothes."

"You were really thinking ahead," Sarah jokes.

"I had my shorts half down. I went into the hospital and they are checking me out and they ask, 'Can you move your right arm?' I say, 'No,' and I move it. All of a sudden, it just came back. I said, 'I swear to God, just a second ago it was not working.'

They were doing all these scans to figure out what was going on, and my arm went dead again. I had two TIAs—transient ischemic attacks—and then they kept me for three days.[1] Luckily, because the third night I had a major stroke. They don't really know why it happened. They said most likely it's from football; I got a lot of concussions and stuff.

They could see a little blood vessel was messed up somewhere deep in my brain and it clotted and then, eventually, I think it popped. My family was mad they didn't give me the clot buster, but if they had, I might have bled out."

"Right," Sarah says, "An aneurysm would have happened."

"Yes," Russell pauses. His face crumbles and his eyes are glassy with sudden tears. "Sorry," he says. "I just cry sometimes. It's called emotional lability. It's usually one or the other: you laugh at inappropriate times or you cry at inappropriate times.

In the beginning, I was just crying all the time. I was like, 'What's going on? I'm not sad.' It was usually when I was happy. Like when I talk about my life, or my therapist, I will always cry. 'These are happy things, why am I crying?' They told me it's pretty typical. Usually it's laugh or cry, and I kind of got both."

"I was actually going to ask you," Sarah says, "Did you learn strategies to manage that?"

"In the beginning, it was really tough for me because I really didn't understand it. They did give me some strategies. Like they said, 'OK, step back and take a deep breath.' And I forget which way it is, but when you laugh at the wrong time you exhale and when you cry at the wrong time you inhale. When it happens to me, I notice I inhale quickly. Maybe I have to work that out and breathe. But it just got better over time, and I cared less. I'm like, 'I don't care.'"

---

1. "A transient ischemic attack (TIA) is like a stroke producing similar symptoms, but usually lasting only a few minutes and causing no permanent damage …. A transient ischemic attach can serve both as a warning and an opportunity, a warning of an impending stroke and an opportunity to take steps to prevent it" (para. 1). https://www.mayoclinic.org/diseases-conditions/transient-ischemic-attack/symptoms-causes/syc-20355679

"When you met us today," Sarah says, "you gave us a heads up."

"It really shocks people," Russell says. "They see a guy—younger guy, fine—and for no real reason … I warn everybody.

They did give me strategies in this community re-entry program—strategies for getting back to life. Part of that is, your friends are going to notice differences, especially if you haven't seen them in a while and they haven't heard the news that something happened."

"And it's shocking for them," Sarah says.

"Yes, and I just like to have fun and laugh about it." Russell pauses. "The one thing I always try to tell people is, when you suffer something bad like this, you get therapy—you get every kind of therapy, doctors, nurses. They'll give you drugs if you're sad. Everything. But your family gets nothing."

"I go to talk to stroke survivors and I'm like, 'Don't get angry.'" Russell's face transforms again as he chokes down another sob. "Be as nice as you can. Don't take it out on your family. These people are doing all this stuff for you and they're not getting help and it's so hard on them. You have to deal with it, but you have to kind of do it lightly. And that's why laughter is so good. They need to release those feelings too, so, laughing or crying, it's kind of a release. I've never really cried before; it feels kind of good to get it out."

"Now you have a reason to, right?" Sarah says, "Especially as a guy."

"Yes, exactly. I have spent my whole life trying not to cry, and so it was kind of relief to say, 'Hey, it's my brain. I can't help it.'"

"Everyone needs that excuse," Patricia adds.

"The more I do it, friends would open up to me like, 'I didn't have a stroke and I cry sometimes.'"

***

"I used to go out to the VA to speak to these marines that were injured, and they were crying," Bill says, gesturing toward the packets of typed stories he's brought us. "They couldn't stand it. One colonel, he says 'I can't cry in front of my men. I can't cry. Why am I crying?'

'I don't hate crying,' I told the colonel. 'I never got to cry for all these years. Why don't you just enjoy it? Why don't you just have fun with it? Why not? It's just part of laughing.'"

CLOSING REFLECTIONS

"People don't even wanna see you when they're eating." Charlie's heart-breaking refrain vividly illustrates the doubly stigmatizing impact of ableism and ageism. For many stroke survivors, the shame and embarrassment associated with their altered physical state is stifling. Loath to receive the pitying looks of others, stroke survivors nevertheless gaze at themselves with self-pity and self-loathing, repeating the merciless mantra: "why me?" While Bill describes vanity as an impetus for his recovery, he also tells us it's the same force that impels so many stroke survivors to "hide under the covers."

These feelings of shame and self-loathing may be particularly strong for men, whose sense of masculine identity is often so closely tied to the physical attributes of strength, endurance, and mobility. For some stroke survivors, symptoms like emotional lability compound this identity threat, eroding their ability to conform to the cultural mandate, "boys do not cry." The consequences are frustration, suicidal ideation, anger, and aggression—often directed at family members and caregivers.

Bill and Russell's stories of recovery highlight the ways in which post-stroke resilience is tied to their ability to reimagine what it means to be masculine. Both men begin to recognize that emotional lability can be embraced as a liberating gift. Claiming a brain injury provides permission to express emotions that they would have otherwise bottled up. Friends participate in this process. For instance, Russell describes how his friends laugh with him at times when his emotional outbursts would otherwise be embarrassing. They use Russell's freely flowing tears as an excuse to claim their own emotional experiences.

Similarly, Charlie emphasizes the idea that Bill's ability to recover can be partially explained by the fact that he had friends who "made him comfortable with who he was at that time." In fact, Charlie's approach to supporting Bill is an extension of their very masculine style of friendship. Charlie transforms recovery into a series of challenges, dares, and "risks," taking a gleeful pleasure in nearly catapulting Bill from his wheelchair and prompting the hospital staff to require seat belts. Rather than disrupting their racquetball-centered relationship, Bill's stroke recovery becomes a new context for friendly competition. Now, as Charlie contends with his own health challenges, he and Bill bond by recalling Charlie's ruthlessness on the court and Bill's "womanizing" ways. As we continue to explore Bill's life, we'll take a closer look at the ways in which friendship, humor, and sport intertwine in his story of recovery.

CHAPTER 6

"Hello! Come on in!" Melanie's bright soprano greets us through the front door of her Point Loma home. A blond bob frames her delicate Nordic features and sparking blue eyes. Her slim figure radiates a sense of youthful energy, clad in khaki shorts, a white t-shirt, and a red-and-white checked vest. Bill has brought us here to meet Mel and her husband, Professor Tom Gillette, Emeritus Faculty in Sociology at San Diego State University. They've managed to remain friends for over 50 years—ever since Tom took that swig from the milk carton in Bill's fridge.

Melanie ushers us into her eclectic home—a tiny beachside bungalow from the 1950s. Melanie and Tom have expanded it over the years, adding an oddly short, steep staircase to access a series of loft-like rooms built into the hillside. We gather in the kitchen. Festive white string lights wrap along the wooden beams of its slanted roof, and a colorful, Mexican-style tablecloth decorates the high kitchen counter. There is a tantalizing spread laid out for us—several bottles of wine, bowls with chips and salsa, thick slices of Italian bread, a platter of meat and cheese, and a spinach pie create the mood that we are joining old friends for a fun evening together.

Melanie pushes Tom into the room; he is 88-years-old, has recently returned from the hospital, and currently relies on a wheelchair for mobility. His eyes look tired but alert beneath a thick thatch of steel-gray hair; he moves his argyle, sock-covered legs out of the way as he and Mel maneuver into the narrow kitchen.

"Hi Tom," Bill says, "This is Sarah, the young lady whose been working with Patricia on my book."

"Nice to meet you," Tom says. His voice is warm and richly resonant—the vocal equivalent of a fuzzy blanket. It's easy to imagine how comforting his presence would have been for San Diego State students who visited him in office hours across his lengthy academic career.

We grab plates, bowls, and glasses and follow Melanie through a sliding side door onto a deck overlooking the Pacific. Beyond the swaying silhouettes of distant palm trees, the late summer sun dazzles off blue ocean water. Mel situates Tom in a chair as we set our snacks on a small wooden deck table covered with a striped cloth.

"We just celebrated Charlie Brumfield's 70th birthday," Bill says as he opens a bottle of chilled white wine. "His body is riddled with cancer, but he still has a good attitude. Over 100 people showed up at his birthday; racquetball players from all over the nation came in."

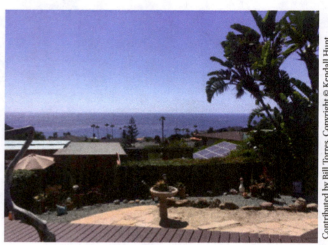

The view from Tom and Melanie's deck

"Oh, my heavens!" Melanie interjects.

"I took the microphone and I said, 'I'm going to deviate from racquetball and tell you what a man Charlie is," Bill continues. "'He's always a hero of mine because he used to come push me in a wheelchair.' So, everyone liked that because that was nice." Bill pauses in his pouring. "Where were we now? I get sidetracked."

"Did you talk about the David Feldman story?" Tom asks.

"No," Bill laughs.

"Now that's a good one," Tom says.

"Yes. There's a lot—too many good ones," Bill replies, "David Feldman taught with Tom when I met Tom in the class they co-taught on Tuesday evenings in 1963 called, 'Determinants of Minority Group Behavior.'"

"Tuesdays with Tom," Melanie quips.

"Tom and David Feldman were both teaching—they were partners. David Feldman played tennis at Stanford. He got his Ph.D. at Stanford, didn't he?" Bill asks.

"Yes," Tom confirms.

"Yes, so he was on the tennis team. He thought he was the greatest player in the world," Bill continues.

"He said that he could beat Bill in any tennis sport with one arm," Tom says, chuckling. "He was a very modest person."

"Because he said that, I didn't let him get one point the first time he played me in racquetball," Bill says, eyes glittering mischievously. "So, he never played me again."

We laugh together as we fill brightly colored paper plates with chips, salsa, and slices of spanakopita, sharing snacks and serving up old memories.

"Tom was off teaching in a navy ship in Vietnam or someplace when I bought the sailboat," Bill continues, employing his usual flair for dramatic storytelling.

"I was at the Gulf of Tonkin, which is in Vietnam," Tom specifies.

"Yes, we were discussing earlier over a couple of drinks that we should get a sailboat together," Bill continues. "He went off to do some teaching at the Gulf of Tonkin and I'm riding my motorcycle over in Shelter Island. There was a drunk guy sitting out in the dark, drinking from a whiskey bottle, and his boat was for sale. I said, 'Can I look at your boat?' I looked, and I said, 'Gosh, this is a nice boat. What do you want for it?'

After taking a swig of the whiskey, he says, 'Well I wanted $3,000, but if I don't sell the boat today, my wife is going to leave me.' So, I paid $2,500. I looked at it and said, 'Oh my God, I'm buying a boat and Tom is not here to say yes. I hope he likes it,'" Bill laughs. "He liked it. What was the name of the boat?" Bill asks Tom.

"The name of the boat?"

"What did we name it?"

"That's a good question."

"I don't even remember, and I have a good memory," Bill laughs. "Anomie?"

"It's a word like that," Melanie confirms, "It's a sociological word."

"Anomie," Patricia repeats, trying the unfamiliar word out. "What is that?"

"Without morals," Bill replies.

"That's not what it means," Tom contradicts, "It means 'those situations where there are no norms.'"

"Well, that's related a bit," Sarah laughs.

"We had a lot of fun on the boat," Bill reminisces. "We had it at the restaurant, The Boathouse. We'd meet and have a few drinks, and then jump on the boat and go have dinner down at the Chart House. There used to be a Chart House in Coronado."

"We won an award for the best performance by an undressed female crew member," Tom adds.

"Yes, we did," Bill confirms. "Every Wednesday, they had what's called the Beer Can Races—they still have them."

"Yes, I've heard of this," Patricia nods.

"We went out and we had one of Tom's students who was endowed with an … IQ."

"Don't forget, gentlemen," Melanie cautions, "This is the time of #metoo."

"She had a high IQ, though," Bill says, sticking doggedly to his euphemistic phrasing. "But she did … she became a dentist, didn't she, Tom?"

"She became a dentist," Tom confirms. "Her name is Beverly Ball. She became a dentist."

"A pretty dentist," Bill adds.

"Beautiful," Tom agrees. "Beverly was beautiful. We got about 200 boats all around us and Beverly comes up and stands up on the forward deck and, all of a sudden, the boats are starting to come."

"They're swarming!" Sarah interjects, imagining boats drawn to Beverly like bees to nectar.

"The Budweiser boat came next to us," Bill says, taking over the story. "They got some buckets and they just poured beer on our boat. Someone took a picture—it was on the wall at the San Diego Yacht Club."

"It was also in the San Diego State paper when Professor Gillette went to work the next day," Melanie adds in a tone of mild censure. "You got a little slap for that."

"Anyway …" Bill deflects.

"Anyway, yes, that's right," Melanie agrees.

"Those were the days," Tom adds, wistfully.

"One time, Dr. Gillette got a call from this heir from Beech-Nut Chewing Gum. I don't know if you ever heard of Beech," Bill says, turning to Sarah. "It's an old chewing

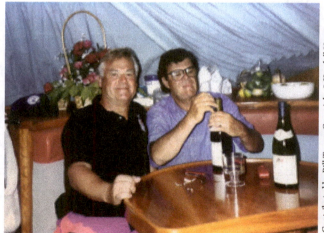

Bill and Tom on one of their many sailing adventures

Contributed by Bill Torres. Copyright © Kendall Hunt Publishing Company.

FALLING IN LOVE WITH THE PROCESS: CULTIVATING RESILIENCE IN HEALTH CRISES

gum brand, before your time. Anyway, he had money, and he wondered how he could take people on vacation and not stay in a hotel. At that time, condos were just starting up. There were some condos in Maui. He asked Tom to do a sociological study on what people wanted in a vacation," Bill pauses, "That's how I became 'Our Man on Maui.'"

BECOMING 'OUR MAN ON MAUI'

In the summer of 1972, Bill was feeling burnt out. Teaching had become tiresome and his marriage to Ursula was on the rocks. When the findings from Dr. Gillette's study suggested that condo patrons needed a local guide to connect them to enjoyable experiences, Tom knew just the man to suggest.

"I got an interview and my new boss, Bob said, 'Well, when can you start?'" Bill recalls. "I said, 'Tomorrow.' I packed up my bags and left—school was out. I flew to Hawaii, to Maui. I had a beautiful condo right on the beach. My office was in downtown Lahaina."

Bill quickly began building a network of connections on the small island. "I was always one step ahead of Bob," Bill remembers. "He said, 'Try to get to know someone over at Lahaina Yacht Club.' And I said, 'How about me?' I met the guy that lived next door to me and he was a member of the Lahaina Yacht Club and he had me join. Usually, it's hard to get in. I joined about the third day I was there. I said, 'Well, Bob, I'm a member. What do you want know about?' He's like, 'How did you get in? How did you get to be a member?'"

Bill intercepted rich patrons at the tiny Ka'anapali Airstrip and Terminal. At the time, Ka'anapali received prop jet air taxis from Honolulu. Bill got to know the bartender there—a man nicknamed High School Harry.[1] Harry got the moniker as a child actor working in Hollywood. Now, he doled out drinks in the Windsock Lounge—a cramped bar at the top of the terminal whose walls and ceiling were covered with patrons' business cards. "On my way to my office at 8:30, 9 o'clock in the morning, I'd stop in there," Bill recalls. "He'd always have a Bloody Mary for me. I'd say, 'OK, Harry I'll see you at 4 o'clock this afternoon, when the lounge closes.' To get to the lounge, you had to go up this little spiral staircase. Harry would always be drunk. I would help him down those stairs, put him in my car, take him home, and carry him into his little apartment. I'd throw him on his bed and I'd say, 'See you tomorrow.' He'd be up there the next morning—someone would give him a ride to work."

Harry introduced Bill to the airport manager. One night over drinks, Bill convinced the manager to hire some local women to greet tourists as they landed. The women would string plumeria flowers together, making leis to place around visitors' necks to welcome them to Hawaii. Bob was duly impressed.

---

1. Accounts of High School Harry remain in local tales of Ka'anapali Airstrip, which was functional from 1961 to 1986. See http://kaanapaliresort.com/kaanapali-airstrip-and-windsock-lounge/

Each day, Bill would meet tourists at the airport, book them a car, and ferry them over to the condos. He'd greet them with coffee and doughnuts by the pool in the morning and ask them about their dinner plans. "Where's a good fish place?" a patron might ask. "Well, how about the Longhorn Cafe?" Bill might reply. "It's in downtown Maui. I'll set it up for you; what time do you want to go?" Bill leveraged his connections with local restauranteurs, ensuring that his clients would have the best of everything—and that Bob would keep sending a steady flow of new customers his way.

***

"Memories," Sarah says.

"Memories," Bill repeats. "Memories are good. Sometimes my memory is too good." He pauses, looking suddenly, sadly contemplative. "We had some fun times," Bill continues, quickly recovering his upbeat tone. He gestures toward Sarah. "She's going to be 29 years old, Tom. Remember when you were 29? I was taking off for South America when I was 29.

"The things we did," Melanie says, pensively.

"I was young and innocent, like you" Bill adds.

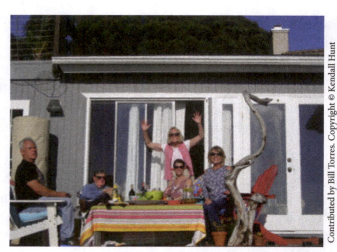

Bill, Tom, Melanie, Sarah, and Patricia on Tom and Mel's deck

"I'm not going with that one," Melanie responds, one eyebrow raised.

"We're not buying it, Bill," Patricia laughs.

"Well, you know more about me than I do by now," Bill responds good-naturedly. "Let me tell you another story …"

SILVER PLATTER SERVICE

"One time, Bob called me up," Bill remembers, "He says, 'Can you score some Maui Wowi?'

I say, 'I might be able to do that.'

And he says, 'Well, there's a restaurant there. I want you to go meet the owner. His name's Paul.'

And I say, 'Chef Paul's Restaurant?' Yes, I know Paul.'

He says, 'You know him?'

I say, 'Well, he is sitting right next to me.' Paul and one of the waiters, Ron, had come over to pick me up. I say, 'You want to talk to him?'

I give Paul the phone, and Bob says, 'I've got these two people coming over and I really want …'

'We'll take care of them,' Paul says, 'Don't worry.'

I said to the waiter, 'Hey, Ron, can you get some Maui Wowi for these people that are coming over? It will be a big tip for you.'

He says, 'Oh, yes.'

I tell Bob, 'We've got it. But it's going to cost you.'

So, Bob tells me the couple's names and when they are flying in. I go pick them up and they're reeking of gold, reeking of diamonds. I had a car for them and I took them to the condo. I said, 'You want to go to Chef Paul's tonight? What time?'

'Yes. Eight o'clock.'

So, I called up Paul: 'Eight o'clock, Paul. Get ready, Ron, have that Maui Wowi for them."

"And Sarah, you know that's marijuana?" Patricia interrupts.

"It's what?" Bill replies, voice laced with sarcasm. "I didn't know that."

"Oh yes, of course you do," Patricia says, sheepishly.

"It wasn't as powerful as this stuff they have now," Bill continues. "But it was powerful. These people, they ask me, 'Why don't you come with us?'

I say, 'Well, that's okay. You guys have fun.'

'No, no, we insist.'

I go with them. Of course, Paul comes out and says, 'Oh we've got the best table for you.' The meal was fabulous. At the end of it, Ron comes in with one of those silver platters and asks, 'Would you like dessert?'

'No, no dessert.'

'We have a special dessert,' Ron says. He lifts the lid, and there are four big joints lying there. Their eyes lit up, and the woman says, 'Yes, we'll have dessert.' They left Ron a $500 tip. I didn't see them for three days. They didn't go any places, but they had the best time."

BORN, RAISED, AND BEAT UP

"Thank you, dear," Tom says as Melanie pours some water into his wine glass, laying out a fistful of his evening medications. "Billy, did you know that I was in the hospital a couple of weeks ago?"

"Yes," Bill says, "But the best thing you did in the last few weeks was eating those spare ribs. I was jealous." Melanie laughs as Bill turns toward Patricia to explain his segue: "Tom went back to his home in Missouri to relive some of his past."

"Kansas City barbeque," Melanie clarifies.

"I wanted to see where it all began," Tom says, "So we flew back and spent a week in Kansas City. We really had a wonderful time."

"That's where you were born?" Sarah asks.

"Yes," Tom says, "Born and raised and beat up"

"I'm unlucky, see," Bill adds, "Tom gets to go back to his home; I don't get to go back."

"Yes, but as a native, Billy, you get to see what the places you used to go as a kid are like now," Melanie says.

"Yes, he was telling us really interesting stories about the start of World War II in San Diego," Sarah says.

"I didn't even tell you that I used to sell newspapers on the marine base and shine shoes for ten cents," Bill adds.

"When we went back the week before last, I was able to see the street corners I had stood on selling the *Saturday Evening Post* and other famous magazines," Tom reminisces. "I used to work the elevators at The Walnuts. They were very high-end condominiums; one family would own one whole floor. I used to work for a man whose name was Herbert Marmaduke Woolf."

"That name sounds wealthy!" Patricia jokes.

"He was one of the famous Woolf brothers of Kansas City. He used to occasionally tip me a nickel, that tight son-of-a …. I would carry his groceries in for him and he'd give me a dollar, maybe."

"Did you fly first class to KC?" Bill asks.

"Yes, we had miles," Melanie replies. "We were going to go to South America at regular class. When that got … canceled … all those points that were going to go toward regular class ended up getting us first class tickets." Melanie skillfully skirts around mention of Tom's ill health, even as the cheerfulness in her voice falters for a split second.

"I've never flown first class in my whole life—and I'm 64—but, one day," Patricia vows.

Melanie points toward Bill: "He took us."

"I took them and my friend Rick and his wife," Bill confirms. "The six of us went down to the Caribbean to go sailing. I took them all first class—I had tons of miles."

"It was great fun," Tom adds.

"My husband and I have been having our own adventures," Patricia interjects, "We've been thinking about retiring in another country, and we recently returned from Portugal. We don't want to be the only English-speaking expats in a non-English-speaking country, so we've been struggling to decide whether Portuguese is just too difficult for us to learn. We lived and worked in Costa Rica for six months, speaking Spanish, but Portuguese is so different! We aren't quite sure where we'll end up."

"We've been going through the same kind of geography," Tom responds, but his soft comment is swallowed up by banter and the clinking of glassware as Bill pours the last of the wine.

PHILOSOPHICAL GEOGRAPHY

Bill settles back in his deck chair and gestures toward his old friend. "Tom is the best listener," he says, "He's not like me. My mind is going 50 miles an hour when you're talking to me. He clears his mind and listens to you. I wish I had that ability; I just don't have that."

"Speaking of which," Sarah says, embracing this conversational detour, "I wanted to go back. You mentioned you're going through the same thing with geography, Tom. Were you talking about physical geography, or your life geography?"

Tom looks at Sarah, one eyebrow raised in appraisal. "I was talking about philosophical geography."

"That's what I thought," Sarah says, "Can you explain?"

"Strange that you would pick up on that. What did you hear?"

"Bill was talking about the future promise of my life as a 29-year-old, and you were talking about visiting the start of your life. So, I thought maybe that's what you were talking about."

"It was," Tom nods. "In a way, that's what I was talking about. I was doing it from a multi-dimensional perspective. I was somehow trying to include space and time."

"Whatever that means," Bill jokes.

"It means what it means," Tom replies.

"What's that?" Bill asks, barely pausing before he continues, "No, you're always in. You're always up for an adventure."

"Amen to that," Melanie interjects.

"See?" Bill says, turning toward Sarah. "You have all these adventures ahead of you, and I envy that. You have all this to do. Hearing us talking about the different adventures we've had; it's going to spur your imagination. You're going to be someplace sometime and say, 'I knew someone who went there.' You're going to be going on similar adventures, just at a little different point in time. That's exciting for me; I can live vicariously."

"I'll just send you a postcard," Sarah jokes.

"That's so sweet of you to say that," Melanie says. "Back in the day, we had the postcard club. Because of Tom's faculty early retirement and great financial planning, we did tons of traveling. We'd send postcards to people, and people would send notes back to us: 'Someday, I'm going to go and visit that place.' Now, we get to hear from our pals. They send us postcards or e-mails."

"Tom and Mel sent me postcards from all over the world from where they were traveling," Bill remembers.

"We always left a photo in a card when we came to see you in the hospital after the stroke," Melanie adds.

"Helping me to remember who you were," Bill nods.

"Exactly right," Melanie agrees. "When we'd go to visit Billy, we'd always try to leave one photo with the three of us in it. We'd write: 'we were here, we love you, we're coming back.'"

***

The sun is setting over the Pacific, a copper orb suspended between gilded ocean waves and purpling marine layer mist. We begin the process of gathering emptied wine glasses and spent paper plates, carrying them back down the narrow steps and placing them on the kitchen counter. Bill pauses mid clean-up, intercepting Sarah at the top of the stairs.

"I've been meaning to ask you," he says, "What is it like to be with some older people like this?"

"That's a good question," Sarah replies, pausing to think. "It's cool being able to just listen to your stories and imagine what your life was like—to envision you in these different places. It feels like being grounded in other people's stories, in other people's histories—in places that I know, but that I didn't know back then. Does that make sense?"

"Yes," Bill replies. "Absolutely. Most of the time, you are just with all of your friends who are all your age, and you talk about things of today."

"Yes," Sarah agrees.

"I think some of this will spark your mind one day," Bill says. "Maybe not this year, maybe not next year, but you are probably going to be married and you're going to say to your husband, 'You know, Tom and Mel did this; Patricia and Bill did this. Let's do something.'"

"You know what's really cool," Sarah says, "You are seeing the value in my future while, at the same time, I'm seeing the value in your past. We are looking different directions in time, and our gazes are meeting somewhere in the middle of the timeline."

"Now, that's a great way to put it. I bet that'd be the name of a good book," Bill jokes. "It always interests me because I won't be around when you're older, but I know that you're going to have a great life. I just know it."

"Thanks," Sarah whispers, tears pooling suddenly in her hazel eyes.

"I'm serious," Bill says, "I wish I would have had some ... All the people I had around were dummies." Sarah gives a watery laugh as Bill continues, "It wasn't until I got in the service that I met people from other walks of life who inspired me to do something."

"Yeah. I think it's comforting to hear from people who've been through other stages of life. Sometimes, you can feel like you're just stuck in the present forever," Sarah tears up again.

"Patricia, come help her," Bill jokes. "I'm making her cry; I've got her in an arm twist. She was trying to beat me up."

"You're so mean to me," Sarah laughs, playing along as Patricia joins them.

"No. We're just having a real nice conversation," Bill sobers. "It's just that I see good things for her future. She's going to be so great."

"Well, she already is," Patricia replies, matter-of-factly.

"I know," Bill smiles, "But she's going to be better."

CLOSING REFLECTIONS

Recounting memories from "Our Man on Maui" reinforces the idea that Bill is the kind of person who could never by satisfied with settling into a sedentary lifestyle. Certainly, this drive for adventure propelled Bill to take a (pro)active role in his stroke recovery process. However, these stories reveal an additional, vital characteristic of Bill's communication style—his penchant for networking. He brags about always being one step ahead of his old boss, Bob, quickly amassing a network of social capital on the island of Maui. Bill is a master of finding the right person, at the right time, for the right purpose. To hear Bill recount his life is to hear a tale studded with happy accidents and fortunate coincidences.

While Bill's talent for networking often serves his own interests, his stories—and his desire to share those stories—showcase the idea that Bill's network frequently expands as he seeks ways to help others. For instance, as "Our Man on Maui," Bill takes the time to help the hapless High School Harry. He forms a routine built around being a reliable resource for others—a routine that closely resembles his current-day commitment to feeding the ducks.

Bill's stories also reveal his capacity to maintain relationships over time. He has managed to preserve a 50-year friendship with Tom and Mel, sustained by a mutual commitment to experiencing adventures together. When Bill is recovering from his stroke, this old pattern of connecting through exploits, stories, and postcards is rearticulated as a means of providing support. Tom and Melanie's bedside photos and cards serve to reconnect Bill to the "philosophical geography" of his own life—a memory map of shared experiences that (re)orients him in the quest for recovery. As both Sarah and Patricia discover, grounding yourself in stories—both your own story and the stories of others—is a profound tool for finding resiliency in the midst of the trauma(s) of living.

Some of this capacity to maintain relationships is tied to Bill's remarkably strong memory. He retains names, dates, and details about the people he meets; these are the tiny bits of information that allow us to feel that we know, and are known by, others. These minutiae become the impetus for connection. For instance, Bill will call Sarah to tell her about a radio story he's heard about a famous soprano, remembering that she once mentioned her love of opera. Bill names the birds he feeds at the lake, remembering details of feather patterns and beak structure to identify "Barbara" and "Philip," and to experience the joy of recognizing returning friends.

Yet, while Bill brags here about his "good memory," he expresses momentary sadness, recognizing that, sometimes, his memory is "too good." When you have a good memory, what do you do with painful memories—with memories of times when people betrayed, disappointed, or left you? In the car ride home from Tom and Mel's, Sarah asked Bill a simple question with an unexpectedly profound answer:

"Do you name the squirrels, Bill?"

"No. If I don't give them names, I can't feel sad when they don't come back."

COMMUNICATION LESSONS LEARNED

While specific to Bill's story of stroke recovery, the communication lessons that emanate from Part One could apply to any one of us in our own recovery from illnesses, accidents, and even the loss of a loved one. The four lessons focus our attention on the value of communicating about our health with our family, friends, and our health care providers and the importance of being informed and communicating about our family health history specifically and health issues generally. The last two lessons ask us to think about the ways our communication can stigmatize others for the ways their bodies and minds change in what is considered "normal" because of illness, aging, and coping with changes in our lives.

A first lesson speaks to how critical it is to communicate with others through any health crisis. Communicating with family, friends, and health care providers about our health is essential across our life-span (Dean, 2017). For example, research reveals that communication with health care providers has a direct effect on health outcomes (Epstein & Street, 2007) and that effective communication can create better emotional, psychological, and functional health for patients (Duggan & Thompson, 2011). In Bill's story, it is clear that communication with his nurse, Susan, played a critical role in all aspects of his recovery from stroke. Specifically, Susan was able to refocus Bill's attention on the potentially positive health outcomes he might achieve in the future, rather than allowing him to focus on the challenging circumstances of his present. In doing so, Susan (re)built Bill's sense of self-efficacy, feeding his belief that, through his own effort, he could regain at least some of his physical and cognitive abilities. Importantly, Susan recognized that humor—often conveyed through music—could be a powerful communication tool to connect with and motivate her patient. Bill's empowerment is enhanced by the relationship-centered care he received, where compassion, empathy, and trust were communicated (Dean, 2017).

A second key communication lesson that emerges from *Part One* is that being informed about health issues generally, and specifically health issues that are prevalent in your family history, leads to better health outcomes (Canary et al., 2019; Street, Makoul, Arora, & Epstein, 2009). Because

Bill knew that stroke was part of his family history and because he was informed about some of the symptoms of stroke, he knew how critical it was to communicate with his friend Sheila that "something was wrong." Similarly, Sheila knew to take swift action to connect Bill to care he would need to minimize the impact of his stroke. Seeking, sharing, and recording family health histories is important. Yet, patterns of family communication such as secrecy, fear, or limited contact may discourage individuals from communicating about potential health threats that they and their loved ones might face (Canary et al., 2019; Hovick, Yamasaki, Burton-Chase, & Peterson, 2014; Yamasaki & Hovick, 2014).

A third set of communication lessons learned in *Part One* relates to stigma, discrimination, marginalization, and ableism. Stigma is defined as any adverse reaction communicated to others because of difference (Goffman, 1963). We live in a Western society that promotes an idealized image of the "perfect" body, glorifying able-bodied personhood. As a result, communication often stigmatizes, discriminates against, and marginalizes people who differ from this ideal because of their older, injured, or disabled bodies or because of their neurodiverse minds (Davis & Quinlan, 2017). The master narrative[1] communicated in our society suggests that, if our bodies or brains differ from what is considered "normal," we should be hidden or hide ourselves (Foucault, 1973, 1995). We see this ableist master narrative at work in the story that Bill tells of not wanting to be seen in public after his stroke. We also see it in the comments Bill's friend, Charlie, makes about how people "don't want to see you when they're eating" after you've had a stroke. Physical difference becomes viewed as monstrosity—a terrifying reminder of the inherent frailty and mortality of the human body. As Lupton (2012) points out, "in public-health discourse, the body is regarded as dangerous, problematic, ever threatening to run out of control, to attract disease, to pose danger to the rest of society" (p. 32). Bill adopts biomedical definitions of what it means to be "healthy," viewing his own body as an object of disgust. In large part, Bill's stories about his initial efforts to recover from his stroke represent his internalization of stigma and ableism, which in part contributed to his feelings of shame, depression, and social isolation (Puhl & Heuer, 2009). At the same time, we see how the characteristics that Bill developed growing up and throughout the early years of his career, as well as his interactions with providers such as Phil and Susan provided opportunities for Bill to reframe that version of his story, and to tell stories that resist the words and actions that had stigmatized him (Davis & Quinlan, 2017).

Similarly, a final communication lesson relates to master narratives that stigmatize aging. The dominant culture in Western society communicates a master narrative of "advanced old age as synonymous with disease, decline, and disability" (Sharf, 2017, p. 40). In her book, *This Chair Rocks: A Manifesto Against Ageism,* Ashton Applewhite (2016) tells us that "as with all 'isms,' stereotyping lies at the heart of ageism: The assumption that all members of a group are the same" (p. 8). Applewhite explores the

---

1. Master narratives or grand theories offer one version of a phenomenon as the certain generalized truth, as opposed to local truths that offer a wide range of meanings about a phenomenon (Lyotard, 1984). Master narratives perpetuate mainstream cultural values and limit our beliefs about the way the world functions (Sharf, Harter, Yamasaki, & Haidet, 2011).

history of ageism, indicating the ways that ageist myths and stereotypes constrain and disable our minds and bodies. She says "the longer we live, the more likely that our lives will diverge from popular culture's cramped, oppressive script" (p. 224). In her view, we need a cultural revolution that pushes back against ageism—we must speak up when we witness ageism in words and actions.

Ageism as a source of stigma, intersects with definitions of masculinity that associate "manliness" with physical strength and emotional stoicism (Lupton, 2012). For men, the physical and emotional symptoms of stroke may threaten their masculine identities, complicating their struggle to recover as they resist talking about their emotional distress or refuse to seek assistance from others. In Bill's and Russell's stories, we see the empowering process of resisting hypermasculine discourses to reframe the experience of crying in front of others. Rather than viewing this symptom of stroke as a threat to masculinity, Bill and Russell instead recognize it as a liberating opportunity to push back against the idea that a man must not show his emotions. In contrast, Charlie harnesses the competitive nature of masculinity as part of his approach to support his friend's recovery efforts. By taking risks in his wheelchair adventures with Bill—even forcing the hospital to change its policy about having seat belts in wheelchairs—Charlie embraces a kind of "dare-devil masculinity" (Lindemann & Cherney, 2008) to assist his friend without disrupting the norms of masculine friendship.

Bill faced many stigmas growing up as a child of divorced parents living in poverty and facing stereotypes about Mexican Americans. But as we know, these sources of stigmas and stereotypes did not hold Bill back in his education, career successes; in the formation of solid and long-lasting relationships; or in his devotion to recover in those first months after his stroke. While at first Bill told his mom, "Send these people away. I don't want to see anyone," eventually he resisted the stigma he internalized, saying, "I was determined to quit bitching about my situation and do something about it." He used a washcloth to stimulate the muscles in his face, singing daily with Susan, working on the *New York Times* crossword puzzles, and finally, with Phil's support, gaining the courage to get out of the wheelchair for good.

REFERENCES

Applewhite, A. (2016). *This chair Rocks: A manifesto against ageism.* New York, NY: Celadon.

Canary, H. E., Elrickb, A., Pokharelb, M., Claytonc, M., Champined, M., Sukovice, M., Hongf, S. J., & Kaphingst, K. A. (2019). Family health history tools as communication resources: Perspectives from Caucasian, Hispanic, and Pacific Islander families. *Journal of Family Communication, 19,*126–143 https://doi.org/10.1080/15267431.2019.1580195

Davis, C. S., & Quinlan, M. M. (2017). Communicating stigma and acceptance. In J. Yamasaki, P. Geist-Martin, & B. F. Sharf (Eds.), *Storied health communication: Communicating personal, cultural, and political complexities* (pp. 191–220). Long Gove, IL: Waveland.

Dean, M. (2017). Communicating in patient–provider relationships. In J. Yamasaki, P. Geist-Martin, & B. F. Sharf (Eds.), *Storied health communication: Communicating personal, cultural, and political complexities* (pp. 53–78). Long Gove, IL: Waveland.

Duggan, A. P., & Thompson, T. L. (2011). Provider–patient interaction and related outcomes. In T. L. Thompson, R. Parrott, & J. F. Nussbaum (Eds.), *The Routledge handbook of health communication* (2nd ed., pp. 414–427). New York, NY: Routledge.

Epstein, R. M., & Street, R. L., Jr. (2007). *Patient-centered communication in cancer care: Promoting healing and reducing suffering* (NIH Publication No. 07-6225J). Bethesda, MD: National Cancer Institute.

Foucault, M. (1973). *The birth of the clinic: An archaeology of medical perception* (A. M. S. Smith, Trans.). New York, NY: Pantheon Books.

Foucault, M. (1995). *Discipline and punish: The birth of the prison* (A. Sheridan, Trans.). New York, NY: Random House.

Goffman, E. (1963). *Stigma: Notes on the management of a spoiled identity.* Englewood Cliffs, NY: Prentice-Hall.

Hovick, S. R., Yamasaki, J. S., Burton-Chase, A. M., & Peterson, S. K. (2014). Patterns of family health history communication among older African American adults. *Journal of Health Communication, 20,* 80–87.

Lindemann, K., & Cherney, J. L. (2008). Communicating in and through "Murderball": Masculinity and disability in wheelchair rugby. *Western Journal of Communication, 72,* 107–125.

Lyotard, J. (1984). *The postmodern condition: A report on knowledge.* Minneapolis, MN: The University of Minnesota Press.

Lupton, D. (2012). *Medicine as culture: Illness, disease and the body* (3rd ed.). Thousand Oaks, CA: Sage.

Puhl, R. M., & Heuer, C. A. (2009). The stigma of obesity: A review and update. *Obesity, 17,* 941–964.

Sharf, B. F. (2017). Communicating health through narratives. In J. Yamasaki, P. Geist-Martin, & B. F. Sharf (Eds.), *Storied health communication: Communicating personal, cultural, and political complexities* (pp. 29–52). Long Gove, IL: Waveland.

Sharf, B. F., Harter, L. M., Yamasaki, J., & Haidet, P. (2011). Narrative turns epic: Continuing developments in health narrative scholarship. In T. L. Thompson, A. Dorsey, K. I. Miller, & R. Parrott (Eds.), *Handbook of health communication* (2nd ed., pp. 36–51). Mahwah, NJ: Erlbaum.

Street, R. L., Jr., Makoul, G., Arora, N. K., & Epstein, R. M. (2009). How does communication heal? Pathways linking clinician–patient communication to health outcomes. *Patient Education and Counseling, 74,* 295–301.

Yamasaki, J., & Hovick, S. R. (2014). "That was grown folks' business": Narrative reflection and response in older adults' family health history communication. *Health Communication, 30,* 221–230.

PART 2

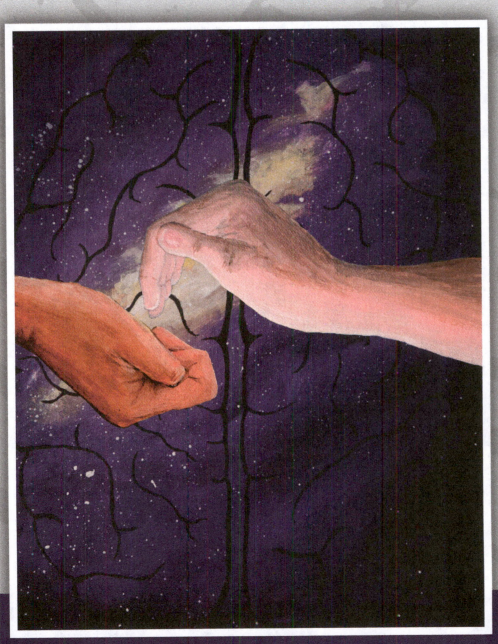

"Their story, yours, mine—it's what we all carry with us on this trip we take, and we owe it to each other to respect our stories and learn from them. Such a respect for narrative as everyone's rock bottom capacity, but also as the universal gift, to be shared with others, seemed altogether fitting." (p. 30)
　　　　　　　　　　　　—Robert Coles, *The Call of Stories* (1989)

"If you want the story, you've got to get inside the heart of it." (p. 23)
　　—Snow scientist Ed Adams, on learning how to predict avalanches by
setting them off and then putting himself directly into their paths so
that he is buried alive (*Newsweek*, December 16, 2002)

"Only thing you ever own is a story. Better make it a good one."
　　　—"The Grover" played by Hugh Jackman in Baz Luhrmann's
(director, writer, producer) *Australia* (2008;
Twentieth Century Fox Film Corporation).

In Part One, we learned about the early years of Bill's life and the characteristics that facilitated his initial process of recovering from the stroke. These characteristics continue to show up in Part Two. In Chapter 7, we learn about turning point moments that contributed to Bill's persistent desire to recover. In Chapter 8, we observe how Bill's love of racquetball not only contributed to his athletic identity, but also connected Bill to a group of friends who would support him after his stroke. In Chapter 9, we become immersed in Bill's circle of friends and begin to understand how reciprocal his friendships are. We see his career take off in Chapter 10 as he discovers his forte as a salesman. Finally, in Chapter 11, we follow Bill as he moves from one coincidence to another, making the most of the opportunities that come his way. All in all, Part Two offers a more well-rounded understanding of how the characteristics Bill has developed throughout his life contributed to his resilience, and to his determination to share his stroke survivor story.

CHAPTER 7

The phone rings in the middle of a family gathering at Patricia's home; Bill is calling. She is tempted to answer it, but restrains herself—she knows that every phone call with Bill requires enough time to listen to a great story. The next day in the car with her husband, J.C., Patricia plays Bill's voicemail: "Hi Patricia, good to hear your voice, even if it is a recording. Just driving back home. I'm on a new mission. I'll have to tell you about it. You know I always want something new to do. Anyway, I hope things are going well. Hello to J.C. and I will hope to talk to ya soon. Bye."

Anxious to hear about his latest exploit, Patricia dials Bill's number. The familiar ringtone is a combination of quacking ducks and jazzy piano music—a custom soundtrack that costs Bill $1.99 year.

"Well, hello there. How's it going?" Bill sings.

"Great, just out and about on a few errands," Patricia says, putting the phone on speaker so that her husband can hear the conversation. She glances at J.C.—eyes prepping him to listen for yet another entertaining Bill story—and speaks toward the cell phone perched in its plastic dashboard holder. "I couldn't wait to hear about the new mission you're on. What is it?'

"Well, guess what? I started a new exercise routine. It's called 9Round. It's a fitness gym focused on boxing. I love it. You work on your whole body with boxing and other exercises and you do it in 30 minutes. I love it. You would love it Patricia. And there's a trainer right there to help you." Bill's words tumble through the speaker phone in a breathless rush of excitement.

"That sounds great. How many people are in the class?"

"It's not a class, it's a circuit. When I go, there are only a few people there and the trainer helps me. In fact, I have been going six days a week for over 26 days straight. They even had someone come in and interview me because I guess I am the oldest one there."

Patricia and J.C. laugh at the thrill in Bill's voice. Getting interviewed for going to the gym is the kind of larger-than-life experience that seems somehow normal for a charismatic person like Bill.

How can it be that this energy-filled gym rat is 80-something? He seems more like he's in his 60s or early 70s—always on the move visiting friends, pet sitting, feeding the ducks, and volunteering to help others. Listening to him talk about his newest fitness routine, it is difficult to reconcile the Bill of today with the image of post-stroke Bill, captured in those neatly typed, blue Calibri packets he's given us. When Patricia returns home from her errands, she rereads one of these accounts, seeking to understand a moment that contributed to Bill's unflagging drive:

A pivotal point in my healing came about the third week as part of my therapy. I was asked if I wanted to have lunch off the hospital grounds. My immediate reply was NO. I wasn't ready to be seen. After some thinking, I recalled the time I was watching TV during some Awards Show. Kirk Douglas, a stroke survivor, went on stage and gave a speech before millions. He was my hero. If Mr. Douglas could speak to millions of viewers, it's the least I could do go out and see a few people. I immediately called the therapist and agreed to have lunch. Thanks, Mr. Douglas." Bill had watched Douglas struggle through his acceptance speech for an honorary Oscar, less than two months after suffering a stroke. And Douglas wrote about how families can support stroke survivors in his memoir, *My Stroke of Luck* (2002) and it was featured in NIH Medline Plus (2007).

***

"OK, let's get started here," Sarah looks at Patricia and then at Bill. It is an unusually blustery and rainy 50-degree day in San Diego. Patricia prepares a pot of hot coffee and sets out bowls of fruit. Our goal today is to learn more about how Bill persisted on the road through recovery in the weeks and months after the stroke. It's clear that Bill is a glass-is-half-full kind of person. But it takes much more than a positive attitude to make a full recovery from the paralysis of a severe stroke. Today, we probe further as we munch on strawberries and grapes and listen to the wind whipping through the palm trees, right outside the window.

"Tell us about your recovery process Bill," Sarah presses. "What moments stand out in your mind?"

FINDING A RHYTHM: THE MUSIC OF RECOVERY

"Music played an important part in my therapy," Bill explains. "I remember a country singer, Mel Tillis. He was a stutterer when speaking, but his stuttering would disappear when he sang. The left side of the brain is for speech and the right side was for singing. My brain was damaged on the left side—it should have been the right, because my singing is terrible!" Sarah laughs, imagining fellow patients plugging their ears to block out Bill's off-key warbling. "Anyway, Susan and I would serenade everyone two or three times a day."

"My speech was improving," Bill continues. "But the thing is, no one says 'okay, we are going to work on this word today.' So, you have to come up with your own plan. You have to tell yourself, 'OK, say *sure, sure, sure*. Say it again: *sure, sure, sure*.' You have to just inundate yourself with words. Then, maybe in the next week, work on one other word. And you have to do that," Bill emphasizes, "because that speech therapist comes in for half hour and then they are gone."

***

For Bill, regaining his speech was a major goal of recovery. One other essential aspect of Bill's recovery was regaining control of his leg and foot so that he could walk without assistance from an AFO (ankle-foot orthosis). Once again, Bill turned to music for rehabilitation inspiration. He provided us with a vivid example of this strategy in another one of his typed accounts, entitled "Tap Dancing." It begins three days into Bill's stay in the Intensive Care Unit:

"When I was finally alone, I started to think, *What can I imagine to help with my sanity?* I don't know why, but I thought of Fred Astaire dancing. And then I thought of Donald O'Connor doing the silly dance in the movie, "Singing in the Rain." Right then, a young intern, April, came in to ask me a few questions. I immediately mumbled to her, "Can you tap dance?" After she understood what I was saying, her answer was "yes." I asked her if she would tap dance for me? So, she danced. It brought a smile to my face and we enjoyed a little laughter. It felt good to laugh. In my best articulated mumbles, I said, "Someday I'll tap dance with you."

For twelve months, I would sit, close my eyes, and inside my brain, I would tap my foot to music, using visualization. It paid off. What a cause for celebration when my foot finally came up! Twelve months, but it was worth it.

Fast forward two years. I am almost in full recovery. I was at the Veteran's Hospital to speak to a group of stroke survivors. I was walking down the crowded hallway when I spied April coming toward me. She screamed, "Mr. Torres you're walking!" We immediately hugged and happily cried. We shed our embrace and we tap danced (well she tapped, and I danced).

These small victories—actually fantastic milestones—gave me the impetus to continue my recovery."

PRACTICE IS THE "KEY"

We pause for a moment, glancing out of the window to watch the palm trees bend in the wind. They look as if their fronded tops might snap off at any moment. "You're like these trees, Bill," Patricia chuckles. "You hang on, you persevere. You tell yourself, 'I've got to keep working on that.'"

Contributed by Bill Torres. Copyright © Kendall Hunt Publishing Company.

"Your friend Randy told us a story about how you used to put a key into a lock 30 times in a row," Sarah adds. "How did you come up with these things? You've basically created a regimen for yourself—daily practices."

"Well, my doorknob, you have to put the key in the lock and the lock is on the right side—the side affected by my stroke," Bill explains. "I'd put the key in there, turn it, take it out, put it back in. I'll do it ten times. Then, I'd unlock it and go in. Next time I came out, I'd do ten more times." Bill looks at Sarah but demonstrates as if the door is right in front of her.

"Did you just find these things in a moment of thinking *this is a thing I can do to practice*?" she asks.

"Well let's see. If that chair is right there. Let's put that chair there." Bill is standing now and pushes one of the dining room chairs in front of him. "You want to learn to go around the chair. But as a stroke survivor, I had to re-learn how my body does that. You just practice it. I played three to four hours of racquetball a day, and I got it in my mind: if you are going to be better, you better practice, practice, practice."

***

Bill frequently describes gaps of support in the recovery process. Stroke survivors who return to their homes may not be able to get transportation to out-patient rehab. Health care providers may not have the time or the imagination to assist a patient in making the next steps (both figuratively and literally) in their recovery journey. Bill noted with frustration that the protocol for stroke rehab was to help the patient to become functional—to be able to button their shirt, to feed themselves, to be able to use the restroom on their own. For Bill, regaining these basic functions was not enough. So, he innovated; Bill developed his own training regimen by transforming household objects into rehab equipment. Bill's initial focus was his right hand. His curled fingers were a continual visual reminder of the brain injury he had endured. Bill slept with his hand sandwiched between heavy books, hoping that the weight would flatten his unruly fingers into submission. He instructed his mother to tape his fingers to wooden tongue depressors, splinting them in place. He threaded each finger through the middle of one of his mother's plastic hair curlers, willing his wayward digits to remember how they once wiggled and straightened with ease.

One of the philosophies that Bill mentions over and over is the idea that time goes by anyway, so you might as well put that time to good use. But the problem, as Bill sees it, is that many stroke survivors give up on themselves in the midst of the painstakingly slow process of recovery. While a stroke survivor might fixate on questions like "When am I going to be normal again?" and "When am I going to reach my goal?" they might not follow through on completing the tiny, repetitive tasks that improvement requires. In contrast, Bill viewed every moment and every movement as a potentially vital investment in getting better.

"So, what if you work out for one minute with your finger?" Bill asks. "Maybe in two years, it will move. Maybe in three years, it will move. Maybe in five years," he shrugs, "you're still going to be around. And this is key," Bill emphasizes, "It's like a diet—very, very difficult. Some people cannot discipline themselves to do the repetition. You've got to do it one day at a time. Today, I completed it. Tomorrow morning you, start over. I'm going to complete it. You don't know where you're going to be a week from now or two weeks from now. You might be winning the Nobel Prize."

DON'T PUT UP BARRIERS FOR YOURSELF

One of the problems that comes up for many stroke survivors in their recovery is the tendency for them to rely on family and friends to do things for them, particularly as loved ones quickly intervene to provide support when the person appears to be struggling. While family or friends act with the best of intentions, their intervention means that the stroke survivor may not learn how to do things for themselves.

"If I had a tip?" Bill advises, "Do what your doctor says. Do what your therapist says. Get added therapy and work your ass off. Make it a challenge. Give yourself little goals: I'm going to move my finger in two months. If it doesn't happen, just go, 'OK, has to be three months now.' Mine took eight months, but I worked at it. Don't let it stop you. Don't put up barriers for yourself. That's what most people do—they put up a barrier. They say, 'It's tiresome work,' and they give up. Then it remains that way for the rest of their life."

As Bill met his initial "little goals" of recovery, he began replacing them with larger ones. What new challenge could he set for himself? While striving for continuous self-improvement, Bill found joy—and Joy—in recovery.

FINDING "JOY" IN RECOVERY

It's a typically sunny San Diego afternoon. We've arranged to meet Joy—the personal trainer who worked with Bill after his official rehab program ended—at a coffee shop near her apartment in North Park. The shop's owners have clearly embraced the newest hipster industrial-chic aesthetic. The San Diego sun angles through the store's glass façade, reflecting off the coffee bar's white marble expanse and gilding the white subway tiles behind the espresso machines. Customers' voices, the hissing of frothed milk, and the rhythmic churning of the coffee grinder echo off the sleek modern finishes, filling the high-ceilinged space with sound.

We've arrived a few minutes early. After ordering our lattes, we perch in uncomfortably fashionable wooden stools around a small, high table, making sure that we have a clear view of the door as we wait for Joy to join us. We have a general sense of what she will look like; Bill showed us a picture of Joy working out with Bill that was included in a newspaper article written about his journey of recovery. While the photo was published 15 years ago, the Joy who enters the coffee shop to join us does not appear to have changed much. Dressed in yoga pants, sports top, and jacket with her blond hair pulled back in a ponytail, she is instantly recognizable. We wave her over to our table and introduce ourselves as she pulls up her own stool.

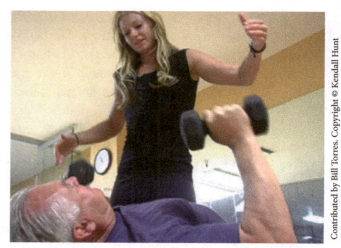

Joy and Bill working out, a year after his stroke

"Usually the first question we ask is if you can just tell us a little bit about your work, so we get your sense of your role in Bill's life," Sarah says, getting down to the business of interviewing.

"When I met Bill, I was just out of college. I went to school for physical therapy, and I was doing an internship, and I figured out that I really didn't want to do it. It was just depressing to be around people in pain all day," Joy begins. She met Bill at the gym when, in typical Bill fashion, he walked up to the tall, slender blond and asked her if he could hire her to be his personal trainer. Joy confesses that she didn't want to do it at first. "I didn't want to take him because it's physical therapy. It's not really something that I wanted," she clarifies. "But, of course, then I met him and he's hilarious and he was so fun to be around. I was just in a better mood when I was around him. I was just like, 'Sure, let's do this.'"

Joy looks up at the coffee shop's high ceilings, remembering. "I used to have him run," she continues. "He used to do these little tiny-like steps and it just used to crack me up. It was the funniest thing ever," Joy's laugh tumbles out easily, bouncing off the store's subway-tiled walls. We join her laughter, imagining an awkward Bill waddling about the gym in duck-like fashion.

"He made me realize that this was my calling," Joy adds, turning serious once again. "I've been doing this for 15 years now, and I still talk about him. I use him as an example of perseverance; if you really want something, you can do it if you put the work in. With Bill, he did the work on his own. I showed him what to do with his body, but he did the work. He always gives me way too much credit. He says 'Oh, you saved my life,' but it was him. I gave him the tools. I was in his corner; I was his advocate. I told him to keep going, but it was all him."

"Do you remember anything about what you saw as the progress he made? Milestones?" Patricia presses.

"I remember when we first started lifting, it was two pounds and he was shaking a lot," Joy recalls. "I used to have to hold his elbow. For leg stuff, I'd have to hold him. In the beginning, it was rough, but his jokes and his personality made it enjoyable and it was great. We did all unilateral, so when he worked his good side, we would try a considerable amount of weight. On his weaker side, we'd have to use less weight. Slowly and surely, his weaker side just became stronger and stronger."

"He used to get really sad when he couldn't do what I asked him to do, and of course I would make it easier. It makes me cry thinking about it now." Joy laughs lightly, but her eyes shine with sudden tears. "I'm sorry," she adds, embarrassed. "He's just so inspiring."

"Everyone we interview cries. He's so important to people," Sarah says, then jokes, "We'll just have to tell Bill that he makes everyone cry."

Joy laughs, blinking her tears away and pausing for a moment as she rubs her forehead. She tells us that she still struggles a bit with depression and migraines, problems that began in those early post-college days when she first met Bill. She offers us a bit of background on how Bill helped her. "I used to date a lot of douche bags," she explains. "I was in my 20s and I was dating really hot guys that treated me like shit. He was always there to give me advice about, 'You're too good for this guy. You're too good for this guy.' We used to go out to breakfast to celebrate all the time. We had a connection there. I got so happy when I was around him." Joy's expression lightens as she describes Bill with great affection. "I don't want to say he felt like grandpa, but he felt like—I never really felt awkward around him. It was very comfortable, and I think he's just that kind of person. He has so many stories. The biggest thing I liked about being around him is he can just tell stories, and stories, and stories, because he's experienced so much. He's done pretty much every kind of work. He's lived in every state." Sarah and Patricia listen intently, recognizing Bill so clearly in all that Joy describes. Joy keeps apologizing for drifting into other subjects and not answering our questions. But she reveals to us what we knew was true for Bill as well—that they had a very special bond. "Didn't he have a nickname for you?" Sarah prompts.

"Yes. Yes! It was Joy to the World." Joy perks up, reminded of this small token of affection. "I think he used to call me a bunch of things related, like being joyful, joy." Her smile fades a bit. "I remember being really sad when he couldn't afford to train anymore," she adds. "I'm like, 'Oh, at least I could still hang out,' and we just didn't. You know, life just gets in the way and I was having some health problems. I thought about calling him. I even called his sister to get his current phone number. We used to go out to breakfast all the time after workouts and stuff. I invited him over to my house for dinner. You become friendly with most of your clients, especially long-term clients, but he just feels like family to me." Joy looks thoughtful, perhaps regretful. "I don't know why I don't see him anymore," she comments, as if to herself. "I want to call him after this."

We pause for a moment, processing. When Patricia breaks the silence, she speaks directly to Joy. "I think it's important for you to realize how he may have done the work, but he couldn't have done the work on his own," she says. "You know that there are people that you train that are not doing the work, and it's not happening, and you're not responsible. I think that, in the same way, when people are successful they just wouldn't be on their own. Bill was at a place in his life where he needed someone like you. I think what you're telling us that's important is that you have a connection that allowed him to feel comfortable, because he talks a lot about not being comfortable out in the world as a person who was visibly disabled. You moved him from a place of discomfort to comfort."

***

With our interview drawing to a close, we ask Joy, if there is anything she would like to add and she says "Even when I have shitty clients and shitty days, I think about him. Thinking back at it now, I keep thinking of his face doing the exercises and how he became a little happier; he'd be proud of himself when he did something that he couldn't do before. He stood up, his posture got better as we did more exercises. He stood a little taller. It was cool. Like I said, he was one of my first clients that I said, 'Yes, this job is super cool.'"

RECOVERY NEVER ENDS

"Hi Bill!" Patricia says, feeling a bit guilty as she picks up the phone. She knows exactly why he is calling; she's been putting off a trip to 9Round with Bill for several weeks.

"Well, hello there Patricia. Are you avoiding me?"

"Why would I do that Bill? You don't want me to go somewhere, do you?"

"You did say you would go. How about tomorrow? I'll pick you up. It's on my way!"

"OK, OK, I guess I'll try it," Patricia drawls out slowly.

"See you tomorrow then!" Bill exclaims in victory.

The next day, as Patricia and Bill drive along the 8 Freeway to 9Round, Bill seems excited to tell Patricia how beneficial it has been for him to do the 9Round fitness routine every single day. "I'm still attaining things now after 16 years," he tells her, "I'm realizing there are things I couldn't do because the neurons and connections are lost. I'm finding through my work at 9Round every day that new things are connecting that were not connected."

Patricia and Bill arrive at the small, dark, square, warehouse-like gym in the corner of a strip mall. Punching bags, weights, and BOSU balls are placed neatly around all sides of the room, decorated in red-and-black designs reminiscent of Patricia's employer, San Diego State University. Music blasts from speakers embedded in the ceiling. "I wish they would play music that I liked," Bill shouts over the thumping beat. "How are they going to get more old people like me in here? We don't like this kind of rap music. Give me older music, like Michael Jackson."

Bill introduces Patricia to Clee, who high-fives Bill. Clee is a 20-something 5'8" African American man. Patricia compliments him on his braids, and Bill points out that his hair style changes every week. Clee laughs, genuinely warmed that Bill notices.

"Bill is my most faithful regular," Clee offers. "And I have to say, his dedication and strength are impressive."

It is clear that they have established a great relationship in the 96 straight days that Bill has been attending. "I haven't missed one day," Bill says, chest swelling with pride as Clee nods in confirmation. "Someone from the main office of 9Round came in to interview me because I am the oldest person who comes here."

"That is so cool, Bill. But watch out, pretty soon all the women your age will be flocking in to meet you," Clee says jokingly as he taps his hand lightly on Bill's shoulder.

Clee guides Patricia through filling out an intake form on an iPad, pausing periodically to yell encouraging platitudes toward one young woman working her way around the circuit: "keep it up!" "stay strong!" "only 30 seconds left!" As she completes her paperwork, Patricia learns a bit more about 9Round by reading the description on the organization's website:

> 9Round started from a place that many businesses do, a desire to change people's lives. Busy parents, owning and running a karate school, Shannon "The Cannon" Hudson, an IKF Light Middleweight Kickboxing World Champion, and his wife, Heather, had a vision. They wanted to create a place where busy people, not unlike themselves, could go to get a killer workout without planning their whole lives around making a class time, or spending hours at the gym. Shannon's martial arts and kickboxing training, and Heather's own passion for fitness were the foundation that the 9Round Franchising empire would be built upon …. In July 2008, the first 9Round location opened on Butler Road, in Greenville, SC …. After its humble beginnings, with that single location in Greenville, SC, there are now over 700 9Round clubs open and operating throughout 42 states and 16 countries, with over 500 more in various stages of development. (https://www.9round.com/our-story)

When Patricia finishes filling out her form, Clee tells Bill to get started at the first of nine stations and instructs Patricia to follow Bill through each station. He points out the signs above each station that indicate what she is supposed to do. Since it's just Bill and Patricia in the gym at this point, Clee offers to assist Patricia as she learns the ropes. Bill leads the way through each of the sections, calling Patricia's attention to different parts of the workout—jump rope, boxing, kicking, sit-ups, and weight work. In a very short 30-minutes, beads of sweat have gathered on both of their foreheads. Patricia feels the telltale burn of lactic acid pooling in her muscles, imagining how sore she will likely feel tomorrow. When Bill struggles with a few of the exercises, Clee is right there to give him a hand or offer some tips. Now Patricia understands how supported and challenged Bill feels here at the 9Round fitness gym.

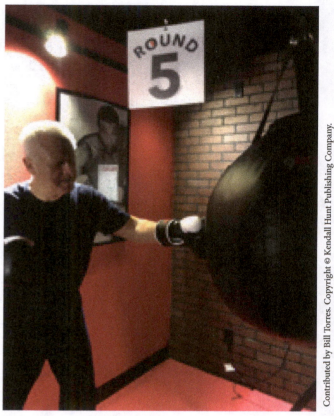

Bill boxing at 9Round, age 84

Contributed by Bill Torres. Copyright © Kendall Hunt Publishing Company.

***

"The first day I went into 9Round, they showed me what to do and I was very impressed with it," Bill says, weaving easily in and out of four lanes of freeway traffic on their way home.

"Why?" Patricia asks, clearly contemplating if this topic might be something she and Sarah would want to return to.

"The first time I came, I broke into a sweat, which I really haven't done for a while. I realized that when you work out by yourself, you work at your comfort level."

"That's true," Patricia agrees, "You don't really push yourself.

"It's good for you still, but you don't go that extra step. And I realized after having that stroke, I always had to go that extra step in order to improve."

"You would stay at the same level of recovery if you didn't go that extra step," Patricia nods, paraphrasing.

FALLING IN LOVE WITH THE PROCESS: CULTIVATING RESILIENCE IN HEALTH CRISES

"Right," Bill continues. "So, I had to go do that extra step. Instead of doing ten minutes trying to do something, I would go 12 minutes. Most people don't do that. They don't challenge themselves. So, when I got done with the 9Round workout that first time and I was like 'Wow, I really worked up a sweat,' I realized there were a lot of things about my body that haven't healed."

"Like what?" Patricia prods.

"Like … You know what butt kickers are? Like, running in place, but kicking your butt? When I first started, the trainer asked me to do butt kickers. I knew what they were, but when I tried to do one, my feet wouldn't move. I'm going, 'Why won't my legs respond?' So, I explain to the trainer—and he knows about my stroke—that there are lost neurons and connections that I am still making and learning. Clee understands, so he had me lay on my stomach and kick my butt from there.

I am finding things out about my body that I still can't do," Bill marvels. "I'm trying to process. I'm listening to what Clee tells me, but even when he tells me, I still forget. So, he keeps working with me. And there are these sequences that I have to remember, like five right hooks, five left hooks, and then five squats, and I will forget after I do it once. So, Clee goes over it again, so I can get it into my brain. It's weird."

"You're not the only one Bill," Patricia empathizes. "At the club where I work out three days a week, I always have to ask the trainer again, 'How many of the sit and squats am I supposed to do?' So, I don't think it's just you."

"Well I feel better now," Bill chuckles appreciatively. "Thanks to Clee and all of the trainers—Ally, Maggie, Taylor, Gavin, Nico, Caitlan, Tony, and TC—I feel special. All of them are really good at helping me with my deficiencies. I had to learn how to do jumping jacks again and I still have trouble with jumping rope. I tell them it is a defective rope," he jokes. "But I used to be good at it. Going for two minutes and 30 seconds; it is really tough when you can do three jumps and then miss. But I really enjoy it because they change the routine every day, and I am learning something new."

Bill pauses, looking contemplative. "I know that I have inspired some of the young people. They tell me, 'I wish I could get my mom to come workout like you do.' And I like that. I hope they see that by working out now when they are young that they can do what I'm doing now, even after having a stroke."

Bill makes the left onto Patricia's street, executing a neat U-turn to drop her off at her front door. As they roll to a stop, Patricia pauses before reaching for the door, noticing the look of squinty-eyed concentration on Bill's face. "I was thinking about all the time and energy that goes into being able to keep getting better after stroke," he says, turning toward her. "It's kind of like your head was shaved and each of the individual hairs are growing in at different times and different lengths, and you're wondering, *When is this hair going to get longer?* You're constantly wondering, *When is this connection going to happen so I have a full head of hair?* Because it goes slowly—millimeters, not giant leaps." Bill's voice shakes a little as he says this, and Patricia resists the impulse to interrupt him with a hug. "My emotions haven't fully recovered," Bill adds. "I try to calm myself down when I talk about these things, but my thoughts get jumbled. I can get too emotional and then I bring back the ugly parts of recovery. But when I am talking with you two, or advocating for others, I feel this sense of connection. I discover new things about my emotions and my body."

CLOSING REFLECTIONS

Every day Bill is motivated to get better, to learn more, and to recognize there are still lost neurons that he is trying to connect to. Whereas some stroke survivors might decide that their recovery is a set point, a destination, Bill sees his stroke recovery as a training—the continual practice of (re) discovering his body's potential. In Chapter 8, we explore the ways in which Bill's background as an athlete informed his approach to regaining mobility post-stroke.

REFERENCE

Douglas, K. (2002). *My stroke of Luck.* New York, NY: HarperCollins,
Kirk Douglas: "My Stroke of Luck" (2007, Summer). *NIH Medline Plus: The Magazine, 2*(3), 7-9. www.medlineplus.gov Summer 2007

CHAPTER 8

Patricia weaves in and out of Mission Valley traffic, driving us home from another successful interview with two of Bill's old friends. The sun has already sunk behind the cliff edges flanking the freeway. Overhead, the periwinkle sky fades toward lavender-gray, illuminated by a massive full moon hovering above the canyon edge on our right.

"It's beautiful," Sarah notes, pointing through the front passenger side window.

"It is," Bill replies from the back seat.

We sit quietly for a few moments. In the stillness, a shared memory steals into our collective minds—thoughts of the moon and Susan from Sharp Memorial. We burst into song nearly simultaneously: "Wheeeen theeee moon hits your eye like a big pizza pie, that's amore!" We try to carry on for a few more verses, but the half-remembered words quickly dissolve into shared laughter.

"Do you see that building over there?" Bill asks Sarah and Patricia, pointing through the gathering gloom to a white structure atop the cliff on our left. "That's the birthplace of racquetball."

"You got into racquetball once you left teaching, right?" Patricia asks from the driver's seat.

"Yes," Bill replies, "But first I had the most magical moment of my teaching career …."

TEACHING WITH THE CHAMP: A KNOCKOUT LESSON

Emerson Elementary School was located on the southside of San Diego—not the most affluent of areas. Most of Mr. Torres's 5th and 6th graders were underprivileged minority students growing up amidst the civil rights protests of the late 1960s and early 1970s. But the school's location did provide one prime benefit—it was situated right across the street from a boxing facility called Any Boy Can (ABC), owned by Archie Moore, the longest-reigning World Lightweight Boxing Champion of all time. When Mr. Torres's students threatened fisticuffs, he took them across the street, put boxing gloves on them, and watched as Bunker taught them the ethos of boxing and the importance of controlling their anger.

One afternoon in 1973, Archie Moore gave Vice Principal Torres a call. "Hey, Bill. Can you get some kids to come down to meet Mohammad Ali? He's in town training for a championship fight against our local guy, Ken Norton."

Bill jumped at the opportunity, but knew that there would be no time to do things the official way and ask parents to sign a permission slip. Instead, he selected a group of 22 students—some of the best- and worst-behaved boys and girls—whose parents he knew would trust his judgment. He called the bus depot and told them to send someone; they'd be going on an impromptu fieldtrip to Ali's training facility in Mission Valley!

As Bill walked into the boxing gym trailed by his gaggle of awe-struck 5th and 6th graders, the legend himself paused his sparring to go over and greet them. "Oh, Mr. Torres, I'm glad that you could bring the kids down!" he said.

"Oh no, call me Bill, Champ," Bill replied, a bit star-struck himself.

"No, no, no," the muscular living legend insisted, turning toward the silent crowd of children. "Kids, listen to this. It's *Mr. Torres*. You respect this man—he is important in your life."

"Well, thank you, Champ," Bill managed to say.

"Tell you what," Ali continued, "I'd like to meet every one of these kids individually. Could you line them up?"

Bill wrangled his saucer-eyed students into single-file formation, watching as Ali greeted each child with quiet messages of instruction and encouragement: "be good, listen to your teachers, I'm so glad you're here to see me." *This is unreal*, Bill thought, beaming with pride. *Here is this great person, coming right down with us, just like he's part of us.*

Archie Moore arrived and made a show of training with Ali, holding up large red pads so that the boxing champ could practice his lightning-fast punches. "Hold on," Ali paused, looking over at Bill and his students. "Mr. Torres, who is your toughest kid?"

"Well that would be Michael, here," Bill replied, picking one of his most troublesome students out of the line-up.

Ali invited the young man up into the ring. "So, you're pretty tough, huh?" Ali told him, handing him a pair of boxing gloves. "Put these on and we'll see what you've got." As Michael raised his gloved hands into a defensive position, Ali lashed out with powerful force—wham, bam! "There's always someone tougher than you," he told his stunned pupil, "You behave, and watch who you get in a fight with."

"Yes, sir, yes, sir," the boy mumbled meekly, stepping back out of the ring to join his waiting class-mates. Together, Bill and his students watched Mohammad Ali spar for two hours until the bus driver whispered regretfully into Bill's ear, "Sir, I've really got to get the bus back to the depot."

"Champ, I've got to get the bus back," Bill called to Ali. The boxing champ paused his swings to think for a moment, looking disappointed by their imminent departure.

"If I find transportation for them, can they stay longer?"

"I guess so," Bill conceded.

Bill's students watched in delight as their hero phoned his trainer, Angie. "We'll need maybe three limos. Could you order three limousines for us?"

A short time later, when Bill recognized that he really would have to return the students to school, he thanked Ali profusely as his students waved collectively, "Goodbye champ, we love you!" The boxing great handed Bill four black visitor passes as he was leaving, inviting him to bring some friends to watch him practice for his fight against Norton.

As the students piled into their flashy white limousines, Bill spoke with each of the drivers: "Listen, here's what we are going to do—we are going to take a cruise around the neighborhood." And so they did. The cheering 5th and 6th graders leaned out of tinted limo windows and waved from open limo sunroofs, feeling like glamorous millionaires as they drove past their classmates' houses. As the limousines rolled to a stop at the school's curb, Bill knew that this was a teaching experience he would never forget.

✳✳✳

"The kids were still raving about it the next day at school. And the students I didn't take hated me," Bill laughs, sounding a bit wistful in the back seat of Patricia's car. "I really enjoyed teaching. But I didn't love all of things surrounding teaching that kept me from being the kind of teacher I wanted to be. I wanted to teach skills like how to shake a person's hand, how to be respectful toward other people, how to behave properly on a date—but those things weren't in the curriculum. Eventually, that's why I left …"

CLOCK WATCHING

Over the years, the dull predictability of life as an elementary school teacher began to weigh on Bill. He took a job as a 6th grade instructor at Spreckles High School in University Heights. He bristled when his colleagues complained about their students in the teacher's lounge, but, after 14 years of teaching, he felt the same bitter disillusionment that comes with burnout. One Wednesday in February of 1976, Bill took a lunch break to drive to Carl's Jr for a burger. When he walked back through the doors of the school's front office, murky feelings of discontent dissolved into a moment of sudden clarity.

"You know what? Get me a substitute, I'm going home," he told the shocked secretary.

"You're going home *now*?" she asked.

"Yes, I'm sick," Bill responded.

"What's wrong?"

"I'm sick of teaching," Bill clarified. "I'm bored. This is not exciting for me. This is clock-watching. I sit in my classroom and think, *Ten more minutes, I can go to lunch for 40 minutes*. I race out the door and beat the kids outside. I can't do this."

The secretary called someone, and someone came. Bill introduced the someone to his students, said goodbye, and walked out the front doors into the brilliant San Diego sunshine. Suddenly, he was free to pursue a burgeoning love—the emerging sport of racquetball.

***

"I was playing racquetball only because I went to a party at Tom's house—Dr. Gillette," Bill explains. "One of the professors there was working part-time at Leach products, which manufactured the first plastic racquet. He says, 'You have to play this game, racquetball. It's really simple.' He gave me all the equipment, and I just fell in love with it."

"You were in your 20s?" Patricia probes.

"No, it wasn't invented then," Bill responds. "I was in my 30s—I was 33 when I started playing racquetball. Did you talk to Bud Muehleisen? He and a couple other guys were instrumental in creating the sport."

A SPORT IS BORN

We balance the phone between us on the arm of the brown leather couch in Patricia's family room, listening to it ring on speaker phone. "Hello," Dr. Bud Muehleisen answers. He is a retired dentist, now living in Minneapolis with his fiancé, Shannon Wright, also a former racquetball champion.

"Hello, this is Sarah."

"And this is Doctor Bud," Muehleisen replies, a smile in his voice. Already, it's clear that he and Bill share the same brand of humor—a witty repartee that closely mirrors the back-and-forth volley of a skillful racquetball match.

"So glad to finally talk to you," Sarah replies. "I have Patricia here; she's my co-author on this project."

"Hi Dr. Bud," Patricia adds.

"Go ahead," Muehleisen encourages.

"OK," Sarah says. "Well, I guess the first question is just asking you to tell us the story of how you first met Bill. How did you become friends?"

"Well, actually, it was through racquetball. We both were from San Diego. I'm 85 and three-quarters, so I was that far ahead of him at the same high school in San Diego—San Diego High. Our dads were similar, where they grew up and everything in San Diego in Old Town. But our friendship started with the sport of racquetball. I started the sport in '69." Dr. Bud pauses, "I don't know if you know about me or not. Do you?"

"Bill has told us a little bit of background about you," Sarah responds, "But we'd like to hear it in your own words."

"Well, going on my last name, Muehleisen, go to Wikipedia. You'll learn a lot about me, okay?"

***

According to Wikipedia (ironically, a source we implore our students never to use!), "Doctor Bud" Muehleisen dominated the sport of paddleball throughout the 1960s. A genteel racket sport known for its culture of "gentlemanly conduct," paddleball was well-suited to Dr. Bud's skills and personality. The unnamed writer(s) of Dr. Bud's Wikipedia entry claim:

> [Doctor Bud] always appeared neatly dressed (usually in white when on the court); he was known for being courteous to his opponents, and mild-mannered both on and off the court. A February 7, 1972 *Sports Illustrated* article about Muehleisen described him

as "Mr. Clean" In the same article, Muehleisen described himself as "The White Knight," referring both to his demeanor and his court apparel. That nickname that stuck, and he is still sometimes known by it today. (para. 5)

In 1969, Doctor Bud incorporated this sense of etiquette and decorum in the rules for a new racket sport—racquetball. He worked with the sporting goods manufacturer, Ektelon, to design and test rackets that would support faster gameplay. Doctor Bud's personal network and charismatic personality encouraged others to make the switch to racquetball and, soon, Muehleisen-style courts[1] were cropping up throughout Southern California and beyond. Dr. Bud became the first athlete to be inducted to the Racquetball Hall of Fame, closely followed by his friend and rival, Charlie Brumfield.

"San Diego became the mecca for racquetball in the ensuing 10 to 15 years," Dr. Bud continues. "And Bill, of course, got involved with it. There was a wonderful club in San Diego called Atlas. Both Bill and I claimed it was our office down there because they'd have little separate rooms for us because we played so much. That's how we really got to know each other. Then, he became a representative for Wilson Sporting Goods."

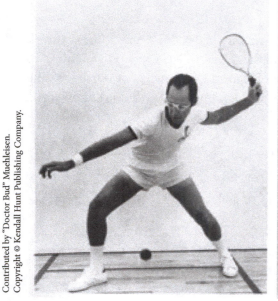
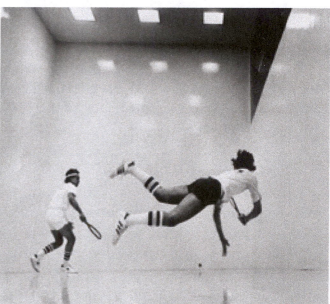

"Doctor Bud" Muehleisen, The Father of Racquetball

***

1. "A four-walled racquetball court with smoothly plastered concrete walls, a varnished suspended maple floor, and an overhead viewing gallery" (Wikipedia, para. 6).

FALLING IN LOVE WITH THE PROCESS: CULTIVATING RESILIENCE IN HEALTH CRISES

OUR MAN WITH WILSON

"Wilson's sporting goods came to me and they knew my reputation in the racquetball field," Bill continues. "I was one of the older guys; I was probably about 40. The other players called me Bones. Wilson didn't have any racquets, balls, nothing. They had just signed the two top players, a guy named Davey Bledsoe and Shannon Wright in the women's division. They needed someone to sign other players—up-and-coming amateur players who could draw people to the sport. Wilson made an offer: 'Would you like to be a consultant? We want to come into racquetball. We don't know anything about it.' I knew all the racquetball players, like my friend, Charlie Brumfield."

***

"Well, when I first met him, he was really a likable person and he made friends with all the other amateur players," Charlie says, recalling the start of his friendship with Bill. "It was really rewarding for me to beat the shit out of the amateurs all the time," he continues with his signature mischievous grin. "And so, I would call Bill over to bring in the sheep."

We laugh together at Charlie's description, seated across from him on a small loveseat at Sharp Grossmont Hospital Outpatient Rehabilitation Center.

"And I would play him and one of his friends—two against one—and we'd have a really good battle."

Charlie pauses to think, then continues. "The thing that was most interesting about him that was so noticeable is his persistence. Because in racquetball and paddleball, which are the two sports he loves, one of the keys was having the physical capability of developing a very high swing speed so that you have power. If you had power, it had a huge advantage for you. He didn't have it. So, what I noticed from him right away is he didn't try to do something with what he didn't have. He tried to do something with what he *did* have. And he persisted in it without complaint and without a negative attitude—without saying, 'Oh my God, I can't hit the ball hard so I can't play.' Instead, he developed his own game where he was maybe the top amateur of the club. He was this extraordinarily gifted player because he used his intelligence and persistence."

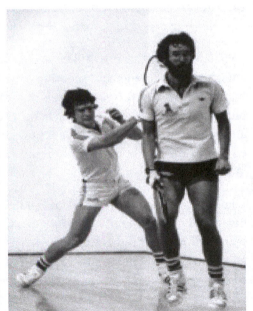

In front: Charlie Brumfield

***

It was Bill's persistence—as well as his charismatic personality—that made him an ideal representative for Wilson Sporting Goods as they tried to capitalize on a trendy new sport. Dr. Bud, Charlie, and their colleagues jerry-rigged their first racquetball equipment by sawing the handles off their tennis racquets. Wilson wanted Bill to help them design, source, and distribute official racquetball gear. "They would send me copies of their racquets," Bill remembers, "They asked, 'What do you think of this one?' I said, 'It's good for making spaghetti. This thing is terrible! It weighs too much.'"

Bill helped to design prototypes using a manufacturer in Taiwan but soon discovered that quality control would be an issue if Wilson wanted to mass-produce the newly designed gear. "I had sent a racquet over to Taiwan that I wanted them to copy," Bill explains. "The racquet had broken strings on it and had some scratches on it. I sent it over there and they sent me back a duplicate. It had the scratches on it and broken strings on it. Finally, I had to go to Taiwan, show them what to do."

Taiwan was only the start. Bill bounced all around Asia, seeking out the best partners for Wilson. He traveled to Korea—the mecca of tennis, volleyball, and racquetball equipment production. He spent several evenings with the Korean titan of manufacturing, Jay Moon Song. "He just wined and dined us," Bill recalls. "He'd always have two limousines, one for us and one for his band. He was into karaoke. We would go to a restaurant and they'd clear the place, set up everything, and then he'd get up there and sing—every restaurant we'd go to. We'd drink soju—which is a Korean drink—and eat Korean barbecue." Bill stayed in Korea for five days before traveling on to Japan, lining up a supplier for the white deerskin gloves America's racquetball players would need.

Back in the United States, Bill traveled across the country as the Pro Tour started up, attending small amateur tournaments and scouting for young players with star potential. He sweet-talked parents into allowing their 17-year-olds to play for Wilson. Bill signed them for yearly contracts of $1,000, plus airfare and lodging for tournaments and an unlimited supply of Wilson racquets, balls, gloves, and bags. Then, Bill shifted his attention to the courts; as each new racquetball club opened, he talked its owners into opening an account with Wilson Sporting Goods. In a year, he'd nabbed 65 new Wilson accounts.

Like any consummate networker, Bill intuitively understood the value of swag. He ordered his own inventory of shoes and warm-up gear, taking it with him from tournament to tournament in the trunk of his car or in his suitcase. He'd ask random players for their shoe size and hand them a free pair, transforming them into walking Wilson billboards. Often, those Wilson-branded shoes directed Bill's feet toward some unexpected adventures.

SHOES, SEATS, AND SUSAN SARANDON

"One time, Sheila and I were in Las Vegas for a tournament there," Bill says, shifting quickly into his storyteller mode. "We went to Benihana's. You know how they seat?" he asks Patricia.

"I love Benihana's," Patricia replies. "They sit you in big groups, right?"

"Yes," Bill says. "So, we sat with other people. This lady and her husband, they were next to me, and we got talking. I told her I worked for Wilson Sporting Goods:

'Oh, I love racquetball.'

'What kind of racquet are you using?'

'Well, we just use the ones at the club.'

'I'll tell you what,' I said, 'When we're through with dinner here, I'd like to present you and your husband with racquets, bags, balls, and some Wilson shirts.'

She says, 'You'd do that?'

I say, 'Yes.'

'I'll do something for you.'

'What's that?'

She says, 'Do you like boxing matches?'

I say, 'Absolutely.'

'There's a championship fight tomorrow night with Roberto Duran. I'd like to give you tickets.'"

"Those are expensive tickets, right?" Patricia interjects, looking impressed.

"Yes," Bill agrees. "The lady says, 'They're pretty good seats.' The next evening, we go to take our seats at the boxing match championship and we're right there," Bill says, pointing to an imaginary boxing ring just a few feet away.

"First row?" Patricia asks, incredulous. "Like, right there?"

"The sweat was hitting us," Bill deadpans, making Patricia laugh. "Little things like that just made it all worthwhile," he continues. "I've always told people, I talk to everyone. You never know what's going to happen."

"This serendipity," Patricia nods, "These new chance encounters."

"Yes. They can happen to everyone if they just talk to people and pry a little."

"Tell me the story of the picture with Susan Sarandon," Patricia shifts gears, referencing a photograph we've seen of Bill and Sarandon in tennis gear. "How did that come about?"

"Well, a friend of mine was working as a prop manager for the movies. When a movie is shooting on location, he would get all the props. Susan Sarandon came down to San Diego in 1979 to the Hotel Del[2] to shoot a tennis scene for the movie, *Loving Couples*. My friend said, 'Well, I can get the racquets and everything from Bill.' He calls me up and he says, 'Hey, you want to give them a lesson and bring some tennis racquets and balls and everything?'"

"Who was the other guy in the picture?" Patricia asks.

"James Coburn[3]," Bill elaborates. "They had a scene where they had to hit. I showed them how to pose for a nice stroke so it looks like they knew what they were doing."

"Were they nice to work with?" Patricia presses, curious.

"James Coburn was incredible. He was fabulous. He came in and had drinks with us—cocktails—and everything. I'll have to tell you a coincidence," Bill shifts gears, struck suddenly by a related memory. "One of my Wilson bosses, who was in Dallas, says, 'I'm going to come out and meet you. I want you to show me around San Diego—show me the racquetball clubs that have been springing up. He flies out and I pick him up at the airport. He was an ex-basketball player. He says, 'you'll know me, I'm 6'7".' He gets in the car and he says, 'Can we go have dinner? Reubens—I want to go there.'

I say, 'Absolutely.'

He says, 'I'm impressed. I got on the plane and I had my Wilson book and was going through some stuff and the flight attendant came by. She said, 'Oh, you work for Wilson?' I said, 'Yes.' She says, 'Do you know Bill Torres?' He goes, 'Yes, I'm going to see him.' She says, 'Will you thank him? He gave my husband and I a lesson, and he gave us some racquets and balls and we love it.'

---

2. The Hotel Del Coronado is a historic, white-and-red beachfront hotel located on Coronado Island in San Diego Bay. Its iconic turret has been featured in numerous films, television shows, and books since the building opened in 1888.
3. A prominent actor whose career spanned nearly 45 years, Coburn was most famous for roles in action movies and westerns.

'That's impressive,' my boss tells me, and I say, 'Well, thank you.'

When we arrive at Reuben's, it's packed. A friend of mine was the hostess there. She says, 'I'll get you a good table by the window. Oh, by the way, my husband and I are really playing racquetball. We bought some racquets for our kids.'

My boss goes, 'That's pretty good.'

So, we sit down. The waitress comes over, and she goes, "Hi, Bill! I love racquetball.' At that time, everyone loved racquetball, see? It just so happens, I knew them! So anyway, the next day I showed my boss the courts and introduced him to people. He just said, 'We're in good hands.'"

***

Bill worked for Wilson for a little over three years, from 1977 to 1981. By age 46, he was at the top of his game (both literally and figuratively), and persistence had gotten him there. Few could imagine how the skills and friendships Bill had forged on the court would serve him post-stroke, nearly 20 years later.

CLOSING REFLECTIONS

Recounting Bill's life as a racquetball player and Wilson rep reveals the ways in which his athletic identity informed his steadfast commitment to recovery post-stroke. In our interview, Dr. Bud emphasized this idea, explaining that "[Bill] was a good player. And when you are a real competitor in national type tournaments, you learn that quitters never win ... [Vince] Lombardi said it: 'Winners never quit and quitters never win.' And that's what motivates him." Bill invokes sports metaphors to describe his strict exercise regimen, frequently recalling how Tony Gwynn—San Diego's famed "Mr. Padre"—never stopped going to batting practice even as the best hitter of his day.

As Charlie pointed out, Bill was *not* the pro championship racquetball player of his day.[4] He lacked the ability to generate the kind of power needed to propel a ball through the air at blistering, "sheep-slaughtering" speeds. And yet, the need to adapt his game to achieve a respectable level of success, despite this disadvantage, taught Bill the value of trying innovative, out-of-the-box techniques to push his body toward maximum performance. "He never tried to do something that was impossible," Charlie emphasized. "He looked for things in his body, and mind, and soul that enables him to excel in the sports. And he really got a lot of enjoyment out of it. And that's one of the things I noticed immediately about him in his recovery: he didn't labor on what he couldn't do. He found a way of realizing that it was possible with what he had—properly nurtured—to succeed in his new life."

---

4. However, In the late 1970s, Bill did win the Master's Championship of California, a tournament for amateurs over 40.

And yet, self-discipline and mental tenacity are only two of the aspects of Bill's racquetball experience that supported stroke recovery. Importantly, racquetball connected Bill to a network of close friendships. Charlie pushes us to examine this fact, telling us, "I don't want to ever take away from Bill's achievements, but he had friends." Already, we have explored various ways in which friends supported Bill throughout his recovery process. In the next chapter, we will reacquaint ourselves with the full cast of characters in Bill's life story, exploring how friendship contributed to Bill's resilience and inspired his desire to help others recover from stroke.

CHAPTER 9

Friendships have played a critical role in Bill's ability to recover from his stroke. In addition, Bill's penchant for forming and maintaining strong social connections has been an important part of his work as a stroke advocate. Throughout the previous chapters, we've introduced several of Bill's closest friends. In this chapter, we weave together insights from several friends who played key roles in Bill's recovery process, exploring what they describe as the nature of social support.

FLOCKING TOGETHER

"One of the things that we're finding really interesting about Bill is the fact that he's got a wide network of friends, like you," Patricia says, enunciating carefully so that Dr. Bud can hear her on the other end of the phoneline. "And we're wanting to also understand what this network of friends believe they were able to offer Bill during his recovery," she continues. "So, can you tell us what you think you might have been able to do or offer him during the process?"

"Yes, I think I understand that question," Dr. Bud replies, "And it's really very simple. Visualize this: San Diego's the mecca for racquetball. The players came from all over the United States. We couldn't build courts fast enough. We were all players and, therefore, we were all working out together. We were all the same, so to speak, even though we all had our own professions, but racquetball was the key. What I'm saying is, birds of a feather flock together." His words inadvertently conjure an image of Bill at his lake, surrounded by the squirrels, geese, ducks, and pigeons who've come to rely on him for a snack each morning.

"Now, when you get someone that's as likeable as Bill is, he becomes a close friend to everybody," Dr. Bud continues. "Bill has no enemies—none that I know of. I don't know anybody who would say one bad word about Bill. Picture this as one of your friends. You're always there for them, you're always there encouraging them."

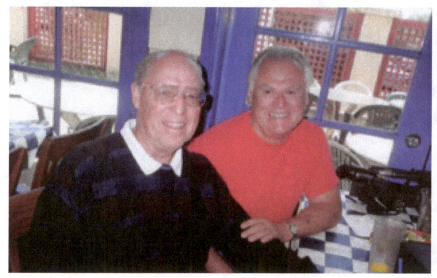

Dr. Bud and Bill

"We got even closer as the years went on," Dr. Bud emphasizes. "We'd go to lunch at least once a week, sometimes with a lot of guys—racquetball guys—and so the friendship just grew and grew and grew. Then Bill had his stroke and it didn't change much, except initially. He was always included, he was always there, so we were basically a support group. We didn't even notice the affliction, but we kept praising him for his recovery. He has to take the credit for being so persistent, but we wouldn't let him quit either."

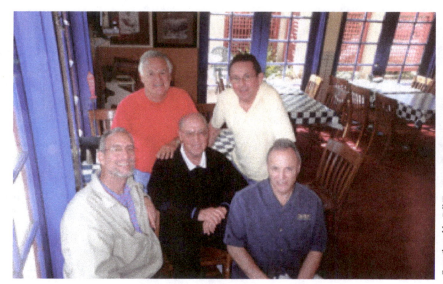

The Lunch Crew: Charlie, Bill, Bud, Gary, and Fred, 2008

FALLING IN LOVE WITH THE PROCESS: CULTIVATING RESILIENCE IN HEALTH CRISES

Dr. Bud notes the ways in which being part of a "flock"—a community of friends linked together by shared interests and experiences—provided Bill with a built-in support network during his recovery from stroke. In talking with friends like Sheila, it became clear to us that Bill is skilled at developing and maintaining his "flock" of friends by staying in touch across the years.

STAYING IN TOUCH

"I was 19," Sheila says, raising her voice a bit so that we can hear her better over the sounds of wind and traffic intruding on our conversation outside Starbucks. "I was trying to play racquetball with my then-boyfriend, who decided we should join this club and play racquetball. Bill was looking over, and he could tell I was a tennis player, not a racquetball player. He was yelling directions down to me and I'm thinking, *Who's this joker?*"

"When I came out, he goes, 'You're a tennis player. You've got to decide that when you're playing racquetball, you're playing racquetball, and when you're playing tennis, you're playing tennis. I could show you because it's a different stroke. You have to get closer in.' And I'm like, 'Sure, sure.'"

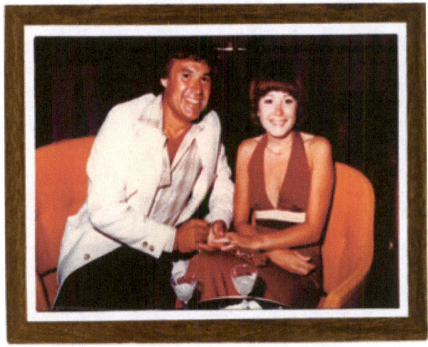

Contributed by Bill Torres. Copyright © Kendall Hunt Publishing Company.

Bill and Sheila

"Bill and I became really good friends. We dated for a little while; not for long because he was a ton older than me—like 25 years older than me. Whatever. It was fine. But it's just like him, dating younger people," Sheila snorts, eyes rolling skyward. "Anyways, we stayed friends even after that, even to where I house sat for him because he was traveling a lot then. He was working for Wilson Sporting Goods, and pretty much supplied me with my tennis shoes and my rackets because I was playing a lot then."

Sheila pauses to take a sip of her drink. "Anyways, you know how things happen—you lose touch, but then you reconnect. Bill lived in Mission Hills, and I'd broken up with somebody. I didn't want to be home on the weekends, and I'd go sleep on his sofa while he was going out on dates. I'd see these girls come in dressed all cute. I'd be sitting there on the sofa and they'd go, 'Who's this?' I'd say, 'I'm just staying here because I had a really bad breakup. Bill said I could sleep on the sofa for the weekend.' So, I would just friggin' sleep on his sofa."

Sheila shakes her head and laughs deep in her throat, remembering. "He's really good about staying in touch with people," she adds. "That's why he knows people for so long; for years and years until they kick the bucket or whatever. He reads the obituaries. He goes to people's services that he hasn't seen in 25 years."

"I call him every day at 8:30—every night," Sheila continues. "We've missed a few, probably not many. Sometimes it's just me talking to his answering machine. I remember when he called to tell me when he moved his finger. I'm like, 'What?!' And he goes, 'Yes, I moved my finger.' I'm like, 'You will have to show me that.'"

"I went to the rehab place, and he's like, 'Watch.' His hand is in the air, and he goes, 'watch, watch.' And beads of sweat are gathering and I'm watching and watching, and finally he goes *beep*." Sheila shows us with her own outstretched pointer finger, giving it the tiniest of wiggles. "It's like an eighth of an inch," she laughs. "'Well look at that, that's wonderful,' I said. Inside, I'm thinking, *Oh, shit. That's going to be a problem*."

"Well, Bill's told us a little bit about some of the things that he did in his recovery that he didn't necessarily learn from therapists," Sarah cuts in. "Is there anything else you can think of that Bill did to help him progress?"

"I think more of what we were doing was just talking about old stuff, making sure he remembered stuff from a long time ago. And I don't even know if it was purposeful. I just treated him like he never had the stroke."

***

Sheila illustrates the ways in which Bill cultivates social capital[1] by consistently staying in touch with friends and acquaintances. These personal habits help Bill to establish exceptionally strong social ties characterized by extensive shared history. As a result, Bill's friends were especially good at accepting Bill's physical impairments post-stroke, helping him to feel more comfortable in his changed body.

ACCEPTING IN THE MIDST

"Well, when he had his stroke and I heard about it, I was in the hospital holding his hand as fast as I could get there," Tom says, seated next to his wife, Melanie, on their sundeck overlooking the Pacific. "I stayed with him for quite a while. He was crying, and I was holding his hand and telling him it was going to be okay. And we talked about how, down within him, he had the ability to heal this. I would make sure that Billy had access to plain, solid research that supported the idea that your mind is part of your body. I listened well and re-confirmed his beliefs that he could heal. I would ask him to show me what he was doing; I could do some positive reinforcement then. And then it was just the power of love—I love that guy and he knows it."

"When you ask, 'what happened between Tom and Billy?'" Melanie jumps in, responding to one of our earlier questions, "Billy told us about the crying and that people didn't know how to handle that. He couldn't watch the news, couldn't watch any medical shows without crying. But also, his sense of humor—oh my gosh, he would just go off! If you tried to tell a joke he'd be laughing so hard. Bill knew his emotions were all over the board, and it was never an issue for Tom. He'd stay in the midst of a guy that would be hysterically laughing and weeping and would say, 'Hi,' with total acceptance."

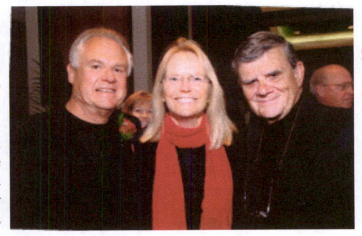

Bill, Melanie, and Tom

***

---

1. *Social capital* is described as networks of relational connections that sustain us and are vital to our health and well-being (Harter, Broderick, Okamoto, Crawford, & Parsloe, 2017).

By offering Bill "total acceptance," friends like Tom and Melanie created a space in which Bill could feel protected from (self-) stigma. Establishing this context of acceptance and trust allowed friends—like former racquetball champ, Charlie—to push Bill beyond complacency and encourage active steps toward recovery.

PUSHING THE PUTT

"You know, one of the most important moments in my life is when I was up on the Balboa Golf Course. You guys know where that is?" Charlie checks for confirmation, squinting inquisitively at Sarah and Patricia seated across from him in the rehab center lobby.

"Yeah," Patricia confirms. Sarah imagines the rolling green expanses, framed by the familiar city skyline of downtown San Diego.

"There's a putting green up there. And this caregiver was there with this giant of a man—the guy was about 6'7" and he was close to 100 years old. I mean, he must have been something else as a kid. He must have been towering over everybody," Charlie editorializes. "Anyway, they had the ball and the putter. And the old man was standing quasi-dazed next to the hole and he would put the ball down and try to putt it in. And the look on his face was majestic. He was enjoying himself even putting from one inch. It was beautiful." Charlie sighs, his face mirroring the serene expression in his memory.

"I told Bill, 'You gotta come with me and hit the golf ball,'" he continues. "The list of excuses that he can come up with as to why he won't try hitting the golf ball is 30 yards long. I said, 'Bill, I'm gonna write these down and then we're gonna look at them, these excuses.' I want him to stretch because where he is, in some respects, he's sad. He doesn't like to come to watch paddle and racquetball. I'm out there watching them myself, 'cause that's all I can do." Charlie gestures to his brittle-looking frame, reminding us of his ongoing cancer journey.

"Bill says, 'My friends are there. I want to be a part of the group.' *I* want him to be part of the group," Charlie emphasizes. "And rather than trying to force him into a group where he's going to feel uncomfortable, I tried to get him to come with me where he feels a little safer. Although it's hard dealing with someone like me a lot," Charlie adds with his trademark self-deprecating humor. "I'm trying to impose my will on you on how to recover."

"So, I want to get him out there on the golf course, and he's going 'Well, I'll shank it.' I say, 'That's not the point. I don't care whether you shank it. I don't care whether you ever finish a hole. I want you to come with me, keep me company.' Once he challenges himself, the next challenge is, 'Let's go watch paddleball and let's see if you can do it and enjoy watching it. OK?' That's what he can do with the other people, too," Charlie adds, referring to the stroke survivors that Bill works with. "It's a lot easier, in some respects, to do it with other people than it is to face it in yourself."

"So, I'm trying to get him to do it. It's uncomfortable, though, because I'm such an asshole," Charlie's eyes glitter above his lopsided grin. "When people don't do what I want 'em to do, I get very upset. And so, I just pick at 'em. Sooner or later, we're going to be out making that 1-inch putt. I can guarantee you that, especially now when I'm in about the same position he's in. Imagine me trying to figure out how to swing with this," Charlie says, shrugging his head to indicate his fragile right arm, riddled with tumors embedded in the bone.

"Anyway, I like helping him. He likes helping me. So, it's a really good relationship. And he'll come to me and say, Charlie, you know, you're pushing too hard. But the first step is wanting to help. Even if you say, 'I don't have any idea what I'm doing but I wanna help, let's start with the 1-inch putt.' Anything can help."

Charlie leans forward slightly in the leather lobby chair, gearing up to share some important idea. "It's like if you work with the hand, it will heal the whole being," he says, alluding to Bill's approach to working with stroke survivors' curled finders. "Anything that you can do to get the people to get rid of the idea that they can't eat in public, or that they can't be seen because they can't swallow, or they slobber, is the most important thing that we can do as fellow humans to one another. And if you look at life, there's always some slobbering that you can spot in any human if you want to look for that. But there's also beauty if you want to look for that. Bill looks for the beauty."

He leans back in the chair, looking at something over our heads. "And here he is, listening in," Charlie says, drawing our attention to the fact that Bill has wandered back into the lobby seating area. Bill hovers a few feet away, not wanting to interrupt. We wave him over, inviting him to join the conversation while teasing him about bribing his friends to say flattering things.

"Well, one of the things I do wanna say now that Bill is here," Charlie says, regaining control of the conversation. "He has been instrumental in helping me move way differently than I did as a young person."

"In what way?" Sarah prompts.

"I just became a nicer, more caring person. And he was patient and helped me in his own way, just like unrolling the hand. He instinctively uses every approach he can to help friends or me," Charlie says, winking as he adds, "and he focuses on the most unpleasant."

***

Bill's friends have outlined the ways that their group of friends acted as a support group, staying in touch, accepted Bill's physical impairments, and pushed him to try new tactics in pursuit of recovery. Bill's strong desire to engage with others was key to both his own recovery and his advocacy work.

WANTING TO ENGAGE

"I just want to say another thing that I see about Bill," Melanie adds. "He sees everyone as his friend. Where most people are guarded, he starts with no filters—sometimes inappropriately. He's interested in other people; he loves to communicate. A quintessential example is when you get on the elevator and everyone's just watching it go to another floor, while he's wanting to engage."

***

Dr. Bud pauses briefly on the other end of the phoneline, considering his next words. "I'm going tell you this story," he says, shifting gears. "I had a bad divorce, okay? That happened. Bill became my process server. I would take him around with things that had to be served, subpoenas and stuff. He was a pro at it. He'd go in and he'd ask, 'Are you so and so?' He'd strike up a friendship, and then he'd go, 'By the way, here's your papers.'" We laugh together, imagining strangers' expressions of surprise and betrayal as they reach out, limply grasping unpleasant paperwork cheerfully proffered by the new friend on their doorstep.

"When someone's your best friend, you do anything for them," Dr. Bud adds, underlining the moral of his story. "And that's what Bill does for everybody now. Because these people with strokes become his target, his practice—his friends. Because anybody he has helped is his friend forever."

CLOSING REFLECTIONS

These excerpts from our interviews with Bill's friends reveal the importance of developing a network of social connections—a process that Bill began long before he experienced that near-fatal blockage in his brain. Dr. Bud's narrative illustrates how participating in the sport of racquetball allowed Bill to find his "flock," connecting with a group of like-minded people who were continuously drawn together by their shared love of competition. Importantly, Bill's social group developed rituals—such as weekly lunch gatherings—that allowed its members to strengthen and maintain their social connections over time. Similarly, Sheila notes that she and Bill call each other religiously at 8:30 p.m., nearly every night. Bill takes this diligently reliable approach to maintaining many of his relationships, staying in touch with acquaintances "for years and years until they kick the bucket."

Interestingly, Charlie, Melanie, Sheila, and Dr. Bud all link Bill's desire to "engage" with others to his work with stroke survivors. At its core, being an advocate requires becoming a friend. Bill honed these social skills as he pursued relationship-centered careers—including a fascinating stint as a traveling franchise salesman. We recount Bill's tales from the road in the following chapter.

REFERENCE

Harter, L. M., Broderick, M., Okamoto, K., Crawford, R., & Parsloe, S. (2017). Communicating health and healing through art. In J. Yamasaki, P. Geist-Martin, & B. F. Sharf (Eds.), *Storied health and illness: Communicating Personal, cultural, and political complexities* (pp. 135–156). Long Gove, IL: Waveland.

CHAPTER 10

"What's My Next Adventure?": From Sailor to Salesman

Patricia's German shepherd/black lab mix, Lucy, suddenly lifts her head from the soft folds of her dog bed. Her short, floppy ears quiver attentively while hackles stiffen into a spiky ridge down her back. A series of sharp, vicious-sounding barks alert us to the fact that Bill has arrived—right on time, as usual. Patricia calms Lucy by stroking her broad forehead; "It's your friend Bill, Lucy. Let's go say hi." The minute the door opens, Lucy nuzzles her muzzle into Bill's outstretched hand and wags her tail with excitement. Bill is a veritable Snow White; cats, dogs, squirrels, ducks … all animals seem to be attracted to Bill, and he to them. It's clear that the same characteristics that describe Bill as an animal lover are the characteristics that were instrumental, not only in his successful recovery from the stroke but in his hugely successful career as a teacher and salesman.

Today, we pick up the story of Bill's life at the height of his work for Wilson Sporting Goods. He'd become bored of his work with Wilson, moved once again by a restless desire for new experiences. In 1981, at the age of 46, Bill decided to sell his home in Mission Hills and purchase a beautiful, 36-foot Pacific Seacraft sailboat. He furnished it with a big bed, a TV, and a stereo system, transforming it into a floating bachelor pad. Bill ferried friends to nearby Coronado Island, Catalina Island, and hot spots on the Mexican coastline. Eventually, he and his professor friend, Tom, decided that they would try to sail around the world—with an all-female crew, of course! The *Los Angeles Times* profiled their plans, capturing Bill's mindset at the time. "I'll be back in 5 or 10 years. Why not?" Bill told the reporter. "I'm not married. I realized I was working to make my house payments, buy more furniture, buy a new car, and knew that was not good enough incentive to keep on doing what I didn't particularly care to do" (Ray, 1981, pp. 1, 3).

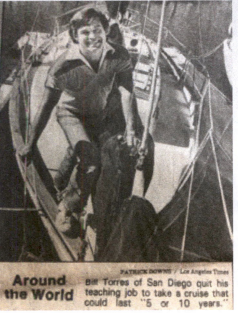

Around the World Bill Torres of San Diego quit his teaching job to take a cruise that could last "5 or 10 years."

PATRICK DOWNS / Los Angeles Times

"So how long did your sailing trip last?" Sarah asks, trying to imagine spending a full decade at sea.

"Well," Bill begins, drawing out his reply for dramatic effect, "it didn't go exactly as planned …"

TAIL OF A WHALE, WHALE OF A TALE[1]

By now, we have learned that Bill's stories tend to unfold into epic sagas. We take steps to prepare for the voyage by refilling coffees and toasting some bagels before sitting back down at the dining room table to learn what mischief Bill got himself into. Lucy curls up beneath Bill's feet, ready to receive the scratches he reaches down to give her periodically.

"We sailed on the 25-fathom line[2] as the direct route south," Bill begins. "It was before satellite navigation, so we used nautical charts, and stayed away from the shipping lanes. That took about a month." Bill switches easily into the jargon of seafaring, tapping back into memories of his life as a sailor. "One day, my fathometer suddenly read that we were only in ten feet of water, when I'm 20 miles out from land. I say, 'What is happening here?' I look over the side and see millions of fish. I say, 'OK, anyone, want to go fishing?'"

"Now, when you throw your line or if you catch a fish, if it's this big …" Bill holds up his hands to demonstrate the length, "you have to throw it back." Sarah nods, remembering a childhood filled with early mornings fishing off the coast of Long Island, praying for keepers. "All the fish were this big," Bill laughs a big belly laugh as he moves his hands closer together, suggesting some pitifully small catches. "We kept some and barbecued them, and that was really good."

"Then, another time, one of the young ladies was on watch. We were just drifting, and she comes back and tells me there's something huge at the front of the boat. So, I went up there and there's a big whale right in front of us. We were going about a mile, two miles an hour. There wasn't any wind, and the whale just kept going on. It was 25 feet from us—we were going to run right into it! I got everyone up and I said, 'OK everyone, start hollering and screaming!' We all were really banging on the side of the boat. The whale sounded, and the big fluke[3] came up right in front of us, right there." Bill points, sitting upright at the edge of his chair as if he has been transported back to that moment on the bow of his boat. "And no one had a camera to take a picture," he adds wistfully, as if wishing he could invite us in to view the whale in his memory.

---

1. Ironically, "Whale of a Tale" is the name of a song from the 1954 film, *20,000 Leagues Under the Sea*. Kirk Douglas—a fellow stroke survivor and one of Bill's personal heroes—played the lead role!
2. According to Merriam-Webster, a fathom line is "a usually sinuous line on a nautical chart joining all points having the same depth of water and thereby indicating the contour of the ocean floor."
3. The name for each of the two flipper-shaped lobes of a whale's tail

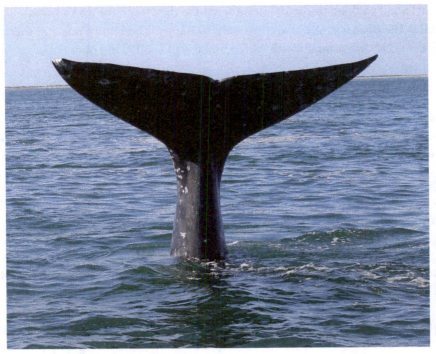

"Another day," Bill continues, "I'm looking through the binoculars and I see the water just all churned and white. I said, 'Everyone up, come look!' There were like a thousand porpoises, and they came along the side of the boat. Then in two seconds, every one of them was gone—just gone." Bill's voice softens, a mixture of surprise and reverence. "That was … that was spectacular," he adds, pausing a moment to marvel once more at the image in his mind.

"We sailed on down the coast and spent Christmas on the boat in San Quetin, Mexico," Bill resumes. "Then, we took off the next day. We were going to Cedros Island. We hit a storm with swells that were 25 feet high. It was scary, and for four days we couldn't get out of the storm. The young ladies got scared, so we pulled into Santa Rosalia and anchored there. When we went ashore, we met a nice family that were part of a fishing camp there. We said, 'We wanted to get into this port and then go back to the States.' I told the father, 'I'll pay you to watch my boat. I'll be back in about five days. Sir, is there anything that you want? We'll bring you food, clothes—what do you want?' He said, 'Could you get a Polaroid camera for my wife?' I said, 'OK.'

We hitched a ride into Piedras Negroes, then took a bus to Tijuana and came home to San Diego. We were all scraggly. We loaded up with kid's clothes, got a Polaroid camera and a bunch of film, and then bought some canned food. We said goodbye to the women crew members. Tom decided he did not want to sail back on the boat, but he agreed to drive with me and a friend, Ed,[4] back down to Santa Rosalia. The boat was still there; we were so happy! The family was still there, too, and we gave them all the goods we brought with us. Then, Ed and I sailed the boat back."

***

"Once all that excitement was over, I found myself sitting on the boat back in San Diego, saying 'What's my next adventure?'" Bill wraps up his sailing saga with this familiar refrain, reaching down to give Lucy another scratch under her chin. "I didn't know what I was going to do."

"Of course! Once again, you're bored," Sarah surmises.

"You know me too well, Sarah. Maybe we should get married." Bill smiles his toothy grin, always the flirt.

"Oh, I don't think my fiancé, Kevin, would be too happy about that," Sarah retorts. Both Sarah and Patricia have learned to play along with Bill's flirtatious spirit.

"So, what was next Bill?" Patricia interrupts the repartee between Bill and Sarah, hoping to learn more of Bill's adventures.

"Yes, you were living on the boat in San Diego, right?" Sarah asks.

"Oh, you're gonna love this coincidence!" Bill says leaning in, both elbows on the table.

FROM FLUKE SIGHTINGS TO FLUKE MEETINGS

"One day I'm just sitting on the boat doing nothing and reading. This good-looking redhead comes over and she says, 'Wow, this is a really nice boat.' I say, 'Do you want to come on board and have a glass of wine with me?' She says, 'Let me go, get my boyfriend.'

'Damn!' Bill adds in an aside, mock-frustrated by a foiled chance at romance. "She brings her boyfriend on board and they have a glass of wine with me and some hors d'oeuvres I had put out," Bill continues, adding, "They're still my friends today."

"The boyfriend, Gray, asks, 'What do you do? You work?'

---

4. In 1984, Ed Gillet completed a year-long, 4,500-mile kayaking trip up the west coast of South America. In 1987, he completed a solo 2,400-mile kayaking trip from Monterey to Maui in 64 days, losing 42 pounds in the process. Read more at https://www.adventure-sportsnetwork.com/sport/paddle-sports/canoe-kayak/gillet/

I said, 'No, I stopped. I'll start looking for a job though; I'm getting bored just sitting on the boat every day. You'd be surprised how often everyone wants to go sailing.'

'Do you like maps?'

'I love maps.'

'Well, I sell maps throughout the United States,' Gray says. 'You want to sell school maps in Texas?'

'Sure, why not?'

'OK, well, meet me in Midland, Texas on such-and-such a date,' Gray says.

'I'll be there.'"

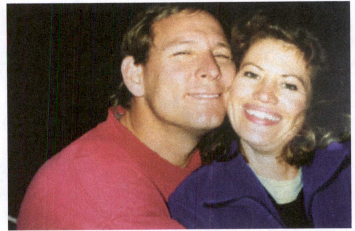

Gray and Joy Graham

"I leased a Buick; I had a Porsche, but you don't drive a sports car in west Texas," Bill explains with a shake of his head, underlining the differences between his posh West-coast life and this new Southwest adventure. "I go into the Holiday Inn in Midland and, sure enough, Gray is waiting for me. He showed me these giant maps they use for schools and colleges. They were geographical on one side and then the cities were on the other side. They were beautiful maps—they sold for $180, so you know they were nice. He shows me a map of California and I say, 'Well, I'm selling in Texas.'

He says, 'Well, we have to get an order, enough orders to make the ones for Texas.'

'Well, will you make them a foot wider?'

'We can do that.'

'Good, because it will be a good selling point—I'll just tell everyone we're going to make it wider, it's going to be bigger than California. If it's not, I will give it to you free.'

He says, 'Good idea.' Then he showed me how to do the sale. 'You get the principal of the school to hold on to the map on the bottom end, then you pull the map up and show all the nice features.' Gray went on one sales call with me and he said, 'You'll do fine.'

I started in Odessa, Texas, which is right near Midland. I branched out each day and drove to hit all the small schools. I would just show up cold and ask for the superintendent. People at all these small schools had never seen a map person. They always ordered through a catalog or something. These maps looked far superior to the ones in the catalogue. And, I always made sure that their little town was going to be on the map, because these little towns in Texas aren't used to seeing their towns on the map. For example, Iraan, Texas was established by a husband and wife—the husband's name was Ira and the wife's name was Ann—so they named their small, wealthy town Iraan. That school had oil on the grounds."

"I don't know if I told you about Kiss, Texas. Did I tell you about when I went to Kiss, Texas?" Bill interrupts himself, checking our faces for signs that he is repeating himself. "That's where Roy Orbison is from," he reports, sounding like a tour guide. "You know the singer-musician Roy Orbison? Anyway, that's where he went to school. Most of the schools had students from kindergarten to seniors in high school all together in one building. A Superintendent, a principal, and a secretary—those were the three who would run the school. At one school, I saw this guy out there sweeping in overalls and I said, 'Could you tell me where the principal's office is?'

He said, 'Well, you're looking at the principal.' In these small schools, a few people did everything."

"I get to Kiss, Texas. It's a beautiful school. I walk in and there is this guy walking toward me coming down the steps. I think, *I know this guy from some place*, and I say, 'Good morning.' I'm wondering, *Where do I know him from?* I walk in, I see the secretary. I say, 'Good morning, my name is Bill Torres and I'd like to talk to the superintendent. By the way, who is that man that just walked out of here? I know him from someplace.'

'That was James Michener, the author who has written about Hawaii; now he is writing about Texas.'

'Wow, I thought I recognized him,' I say.

She says, 'The superintendent didn't even know who James Michener was.'

'What?' I say, and I get an idea. I tell the secretary, 'You go in there and tell him, Truman Capote is here.'

She smiles and says out loud, 'That will be great. I doubt if he knows him.' She walks in there and tells him, and the guy comes out to me and says, 'Hi, Mr. Capote?' The secretary and I laugh at him and he says, 'Wait, what is this?' Then we told him what we did. He got a kick out of it and I sold him three maps."

***

By this time, we need a break to stretch our legs and take a breath of fresh air. We gather outside on Patricia's sundeck, taking in a panoramic view of the San Diego landscape—the palm-tree-dotted cliff edges of Mission Valley, the white stucco buildings of San Diego State's sprawling campus, the distant skyscrapers of downtown, and the distinct curve of the Coronado Bride, rising from the blue mists of San Diego Bay.

"How long did you do the map selling?" Sarah asks Bill, eyes still turned toward the horizon.

"I did that for two years," Bill answers.

"Two years?" Patricia questions incredulously. "If Wilson Sports wanted you to be a salesperson and you didn't want to do it then, what made you do map sales for two years?"

Bill smiles and reflects, "It was just timing. Timing is everything in life. If I hadn't been sitting on my boat and that good-looking redhead hadn't walked by, I would have been doing something else, right?

"There was something more appealing about traveling and selling maps than selling Wilson gear?" Sarah probes.

Bill nods in agreement, "I just needed to change, and I didn't know what I was gonna do. I thought selling maps was a nice thing. It gave me a chance to travel, to see a lot of little towns. It was wonderful seeing these little towns and how they cope with life." Bill pauses for a moment, absorbing the San Diego sun and recalling the baking heat of west Texas. Lucy joins us on the deck to sit next to Bill's feet and lean against his side. He pats her head absent-mindedly as he launches into a new set of stories, sharing his impressions of little town life.

LITTLE TOWN LIFE, BIG TIME DRAMA

"I visited a school district in Big Lake, Texas," Bill recalls. "The grandfather was the superintendent, the father was the principal, the wife was the secretary and the daughter was a secretary—the whole family. I remember asking the young lady, 'Have you ever been out of a Big Lake, Texas?' She says, 'No, but my mother went to Dallas once.' They spend their whole life in a small town," Bill emphasizes, "and don't leave."

"One time, I was down in Sonora, Mexico," Bill continues. "I called it the 'dead deer capital' because the truck drivers there would brag about how often they run over the wild deer. I pull into this motel and I asked the receptionist, 'I'm really hungry. What's the best restaurant in town?'

She says, 'Mom's.'

I say, 'Well, I don't know your mom.'

She says, 'No, Mom's Restaurant. Everyone knows Mom's restaurant.'

'I'm new here. I don't know Mom's Restaurant.'

'You'll just go down the block, you'll see it.'

Sure enough, I see a big sign, 'Mom's.' So, I go down there, have some lunch, and it was good. I come back and I see there's a restaurant across the street from the motel, but it's behind a building. I walk in to the motel and say, 'How come you didn't point me to that restaurant?'

She said, 'That's new here and I haven't eaten there yet.'

I said, 'How long has it been there?'

'Four years.'

"It's just little things like that," Bill summarizes with a smile "You see the charm in these little towns."

"Oh, and another thing about Texas. You talk about gun crime?" Bill shifting abruptly to a less charming subject. "Well, I used to go to Odessa and I met the Holiday Inn manager, Lucy, and her husband. One night, I went out with Lucy to a bar in Odessa, right where the oil fields are. All the riggers and young guys come in their trucks and have a drink. It was two for the price of one. They order a Crown Royal. They say, 'Give me two,' so they get four. Then, they say, 'Give me one beer,' and they get two beers.

One night they had a band and everyone's dancing and this young lady walks up to me and she says, 'Are you here with anyone?'

'No.'

'Would you like to dance?' Since Lucy had gone to the bathroom, I say, 'Sure, I would like to dance.' I go out and dance with her and I come back and Lucy comes over and says, 'Don't dance with that girl.'

'What's wrong?'

'Her boyfriend is crazy; he'll beat you up. You don't know these rednecks here.'

I say, 'Thanks for the warning.' The young girl comes up and asks me to dance again and I say, 'I can't right now.'

There is a guy next to me and she says, 'How about you? Would you like to dance?' He says yes, so they go to dance floor. I'm talking to Lucy. All of a sudden, there's two shots: BAM! BAM! The music stops. The young girl's boyfriend came in and shot the guy she was dancing with right in the stomach."

"Oh my God, Bill! For dancing with his girlfriend?!" Patricia says, voice high-pitched with shock.

"Yea, it could have been me!" Bill exclaims.

"Yes, it sure could have," Sarah agrees, eyebrows drawn in concern. "Did he die?"

"No, they took him off and he was okay," Bill says casually.

"And that's when I said to myself, 'OK, I'm done selling maps.' Plus, I was done with the travel. I would drive all around Texas for three weeks, then I'd fly home and stay in San Diego for a week, then fly back and drive around again for three weeks. I got tired of that. I realized 'I can't do this anymore.'"

Bill stops, a familiar mischievous smile spreading across his face. "Aren't you tired of me yet?" he asks.

"Never," Sarah responds, patting Bill's shoulder, "Never, Bill. You have led such an amazing life."

"We just can't get enough," Patricia adds.

"Well, then," Bill says, "I need to tell you about another fabulous coincidence!"

CLOSING REFLECTIONS

We have learned again and again that Bill is a people person. He thrives on conversations and experiences with others. What we also see in Bill is his adaptability. While Bill grew up in the large city of San Diego and he has traveled the world, he easily adapted to small town Texas, making friends and learning what he could about the culture. This adaptability served him well in traveling back and forth from Texas to San Diego for two years. Some people could not do what Bill did for two years—driving all over and situating himself in small towns, meeting new people, staying in new places, and making the trip back and forth every few weeks. Where many people might hesitate or worry about a spur of the moment decision, Bill jumped on these opportunities. As we'll see in this next chapter, Bill's capacity to remain flexible and adaptable meant that he was able to transform a series of unexpected "coincidences" into opportunities for connection and personal growth.

REFERENCE

Ray, N. (1981, November 22). Sailing off to adventure: A dream come true for many. *Los Angeles Times (San Diego County section)*, pp. CC Part II, 1, 3, 8.

CHAPTER 11

"Is it okay that Stella keeps jumping up on your lap, Bill?" Patricia asks, reaching to pet the gray-and-white speckled cat cuddled across Bill's thighs. We've settled back at Patricia's honey oak dining room table, awaiting Bill's account of life after west Texas.

"Oh, I love it!" Bill pats Stella affectionately. "I really think she is Charlie reincarnated. He was just like this—a cuddler every time I sat down. Did I tell you the story about my $4,000 cat, Charlie?" Bill asks Sarah.

"Well, no?" Sarah says tentatively.

"When I put an offer on a house in San Diego, the owners said they couldn't take Charlie with them. They asked me if I could take Charlie, love him, and keep him happy. Well, you know me. I said 'Sure, I love animals.' Well, it turned out that the other offer for the house was $4,000 more than mine, but the guy told the owners that he could not take Charlie. So, guess what? They sold the house to me and I ended up with my good friend, Charlie. And that's how he became my $4,000 cat."

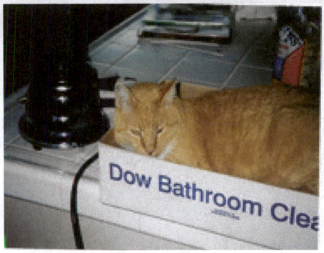

Charlie, the $4,000 cat.

Contributed by Bill Torres. Copyright © Kendall Hunt Publishing Company.

"Charlie's reincarnated as Stella," Patricia says, chuckling as she reaches over to pet her cat.

"Charlie sounds like just another example of your random good luck," Sarah observes.

"Yep," Bill agrees, "Kind of like the stroke of luck that ended my map-selling days …."

FRANCHISING FOR FERRAGAMO

"So, after my last trip to Texas, I got home and I'm sitting on my boat," Bill tells us, picking up the thread of his life story. "I'm walking down the dock and I see an old friend; I used to go out with his sister.

'Hey, Craig!' I say.

'Hi Bill! I was telling people that you live on a boat out here. Where is your boat?'

I point to my boat and say, 'This is it! What are you doing now?'

'I just went to work for Arby's in real estate.'

'Are there any sales jobs?' I asked. 'Let me know. I'm a salesman now.'

That evening, I head over to my mom's house for dinner and the phone rings. I pick it up and it's Craig. He says, 'Hey, the sales guy in California for Arby's just had a heart-attack. They are looking for a salesman. Do you want me to put your name in?'

I say, 'Absolutely. I'll send a resume right away.' At that time, you faxed things," Bill adds, suddenly aware of Sarah's youth. "So, I faxed the resume. A guy flew out to interview me, and I got hired."

"When you say sales, what do you mean?" Sarah interrupts.

"Selling franchises," Bill clarifies. "I never sold a franchise in my life. But I sold franchises for Arby's. If you wanted to franchise here in San Diego, you' d come see me and then we'd sit down. Then, if I thought you were qualified, I would have you go back to Arby's headquarters in Atlanta. We'd sign all the papers there and start you on your way."

"How old were you by this time?" Patricia asks.

"I was probably 40, 42."

"Wait," Sarah says. "You had to be older than 42 because you said you were about 47 when you started mapping."

"Let's see, it was 1984. I'm 82 now so I would have been …',

"I can't do that calculation, Bill," Patricia laughs.

"Come on, come on, use your math skills!" Bill teases

Sarah adds it up: "You were born in '35, so you were 49."

"OK, 49 then!"

"Wow, and you said you were 42," Patricia kids, making fun of Bill's habit of always claiming to be younger.

"Anyway," Sarah cuts in, "You're 49 and you're selling Arby's franchises."

"Yeah. There were six guys selling franchises across the United States. I had 14 western states including Alaska and Hawaii, and I had to travel to all those states. By the time I was let go, I had over 1,000,000 miles on Delta, 250,000 miles on American, and 400,000 on United. I had so many miles, I would fly every place first class. I did that for 10 years."

"You said you were let go?" Sarah prompts.

"Yes, there was nothing else to sell," Bill explains. "Unbeknownst to me, the best type of sale is a negative sale where you convince the guy that he doesn't want it. You don't want the guy to have it because he can't succeed in a saturated market. But, when you tell them they don't want it, they want it more. I didn't know that was a negative sale. I would tell people the truth. I'd say, 'Look, you don't want an Arby's here, you'll fail.'"

"Anyway, the first six months, I sold nine franchises. That was unheard of. Everyone else sold maybe two or three a year. They said, 'What are you doing that we are not doing?' I said, 'I do a little negative sale.' I just ask them, 'What you want in life? Why do you want to do this? You don't want this. You are going to lose your ass.' And that really make them want this.

Anyway, I was very successful. I was good at the negative sale, asking question after question, getting them on board to really want it. Arby's was impressed with my success, so they asked me to do a presentation to the other salesmen.

We were all very successful. One six-month bonus was $63,000, on top of my salary of $50,000. It's $50,000 plus commission, and all your expenses are paid."

"So, did you have money saved at this point?" Sarah asks

"No. What for?" Bill retorts, "What's this stuff on saving?"

"It's highly ingrained in our culture to save money," Patricia responds, lapsing into professor mode.

"Yes, highly overrated," Bill snorts. "I was making a lot of money, so I started buying Armani suits, Canali suits, Brioni ties, Ferragamo shoes."

"You were the man," Patricia enthuses, imagining a middle-aged Bill dressed to the nines.

"Yes," Bill agrees, reminiscing. "I had tons of money, and we would travel. Our meetings were in Jamaica, Puerto Rico, Paradise Island at Nassau, the Bahamas. Our boss was first class guy. We'd always go to the best hotels, the best restaurants. And everywhere I went, there were co-incidences. I'm always full of coincidences, I think I've told you that. Here," Bill continues, "let me give you a few examples …."

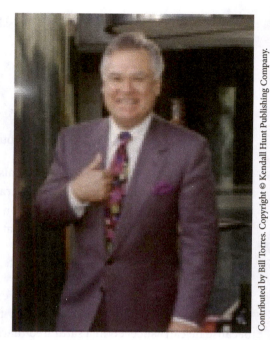

Bill in his favorite suit

SERENDIPITY STRIKES AGAIN

Listening to Bill recount the highlights of his career as a franchise salesman is like listening to a television screen-writer pitch 30-minute episodes for the latest situational comedy. For example, Bill told us about a business trip to Louisville, Kentucky to attend the Kentucky Derby. Bill's boss, Jim, tasked him with finding a restaurant in nearby Shelbyville that might accommodate their party of 25 businesspeople. Before the days of Yelp and Google, the request seemed like a tall order. Bill still hadn't figured out a plan by the time he boarded a flight to San Diego, settling into a first-class seat next to an attractive young woman. In the process of striking up a conversation with his lovely seatmate, Bill discovered that she was from Kentucky. "Our sales force is going to the Kentucky Derby," Bill told the woman, "but we're not staying in Louisville because all the hotels were booked. We're staying in a place called Shelbyville."

"Well, that's where I'm from," she replied.

"Really? Tell me about it. I've got to find the best restaurant in Shelbyville."

"Well, do you like Italian food?' Bill's travel buddy inquired. "My mom and dad have the best restaurant, and it's in Shelbyville," she continued, picking up the chunky 1980's plane phone embedded in the seat back in front of her. "I can call up my mother now and make reservations."

Bill got off the plane in San Diego and called his boss, telling him about his chance encounter. "Everything's set up," he reported. "I've got a restaurant in Shelbyville."

"You big bullshitter," an incredulous Jim replied. "You're so full of bull."

"No, it's true," Bill reassured. The next evening, Bill's coworkers gathered around a large banquet table in Shelbyville's finest Italian restaurant, complete with fresh flowers and complimentary wine. They watched in astonishment as the proprietress and her daughter greeted Bill with a hug.

"This is unbelievable," Jim uttered, floored.

"Well, you told me to get a good restaurant," Bill quipped.

***

Stories like this one are often followed by the phrase "another coincidence," as Bill segues rapidly from one larger-than-life tale to another. He tells us about the time another boss, Russ, an Australian, flew from Atlanta to meet with Bill and to see Los Angeles for the first time.

"Russ, is there anything that you want to do while you're in LA, sightseeing?" Bill asked him.

"Yes, I want to see a movie star," Russ replied.

"Well, anyone in particular?"

"I love Fred Astaire."

"Well, I'm going to set up a reservation for a nice restaurant out on Santa Monica Boulevard," Bill replied. "There are movie stars that dine there all the time."

After a long day of travel and franchisee meetings, Bill and Russ finally sat down to order their food at the popular LA spot Bill had chosen. Bill, glancing over his boss's shoulder at the people coming in and out the front doors, stiffened in shock as he recognized the restaurant's newest patron—a wizened, 95-year-old Fred Astaire had just walked in.

"Russ, look over there to your left," Bill whispered.

"Oh my God," Russ breathed, spotting the Hollywood dance icon. "How did you do it?"

"You wanted Fred Astaire," Bill responded with a nonchalant shrug. "You're my boss."

"This is unbelievable. What should we do?"

"Well, we're almost done. We'll walk by his table and just say, 'Mr. Astaire, I love your movies and I think you're a classy guy.'" Bill asked for the check and a few to-go boxes, then shepherded his star-struck boss toward his idol's booth. The poor man simply stammered, tongue-tied. "Mr. Astaire, we love your movies," Bill supplied. When the Hollywood royal responded with a soft "thank you," Russ nearly died on the spot.

Several years later, when Russ found out that Bill had a stroke, he called him from Australia. "I tell everyone that story," Russ reported, "and they don't believe me."

"OK, keep telling them," Bill replied, "That was just another one of the million coincidences in my life."

A NEW YORK MINUTE

"So, the Arby's gig dried up because you saturated the market," Sarah summarizes as Bill pauses to scratch Stella behind the ears. "What did you do next?"

"A headhunter named Steve called me and said, 'Bill, you on the market? There's a real good job. You can make a lot of money. The guy's got a lot of money. He's got a small restaurant chain. He wants to expand internationally.'"

"So this position involved selling franchises again?" Patricia asks.

"Yes," Bill indicated. "Selling franchises for Pudgie's Famous Chicken in Long Island, NY. I filled up my BMW and told my mom, 'I'm moving to New York for a while. I don't know how long.'

I drove all the way to New York, and the only time I got lost was when I went to cross the Verrazano bridge, a double-decked suspension bridge that connects Staten Island and Brooklyn. I couldn't find the road. But I finally got to Uniondale, New York and found a nice big office; my new title is Senior Vice-President.

Steve said, 'We're going to make a million. We're going to go down to Wall Street. You're going to give a talk on Wall Street to this firm. We're going to get the stock up. You're going to give them all the projections. Then, we're going to become millionaires.'

I said, 'Fine with me.' It was a very good chicken.

I went to work immediately. I sold ten stores in Jakarta, Indonesia in the first three months, and two in California. When I flew over to Jakarta, people there treated me like a king and sent me over to Bali for three days to sit on the beach, all expenses paid. When I came back and Steve asked, 'How'd it go?' I just gave him all these pictures from the grand opening.

So, I was with them for about seven months. But what happened is, the whole thing fell apart. The owner was losing so much money; he couldn't support the store. The stock went down to a dollar. They couldn't afford me. So, that was the end of that.

I didn't like New York anyway. It was a new experience for me to live in New York. The people there are just weird. I jumped in my car and drove all the way back to Escondido. If I didn't have to stop for the first stoplight from the office, and if I wouldn't have had to stop for the tollways, and if I didn't have to stop to go to the bathroom, or at a motel, or eat, I could drive all the way to Escondido without stopping. That's how good our freeway system is."

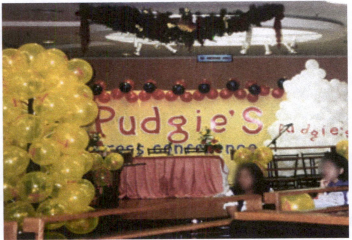

Photo from Pudgie's Grand Opening, Jakarta, Indonesia, 1997

Contributed by Bill Torres. Copyright © Kendall Hunt Publishing Company.

***

Once Bill got back to California, it was only two months later that another opportunity fell into his lap. His neighbor Craig—the man who had initially told Bill about the Arby's opportunities—had switched over to selling for the competitor fast food franchise, Carl's Jr. Craig approached Bill about an opportunity to handle Carl's Jr's international sales in Mexico. Bill took the position to become Director of Franchising and worked out of the Santa Barbara, California office from 1999-2002. Soon, however, the restless urge to try something new returned. So, Bill rented a place in the San Diego neighborhood of Little Italy and began brainstorming new options. It was during that time, in between jobs and with no insurance, that disaster struck; Bill suffered his paralyzing stroke. But stroke, of course, was not the end of Bill's story.

CLOSING REFLECTIONS

It's impossible to know if all of the coincidences and opportunities that came Bill's way were of his creation or just the luck of the draw. However, based on what we have learned about Bill's life story, we would guess that Bill is one of those people that do not wait around for something great to materialize that they make it happen. But how? Bill's resilience and ability to thrive throughout his life is something he creates through his outgoing personality, curiosity about all things, and people he meets, as well as his inability to stay put in one place for too long. Some would call him a lifelong learner.[1] Others might say he is a people person. Whatever the case, his experience as a salesman over a 20-year stretch of time, in four different businesses, offers lessons for anyone who wants to learn what it takes to become resilient after a paralyzing stroke.

For Bill Torres, there is the power of "Yes, why not?" when an opportunity comes knocking. We have noticed that throughout these 20 years, Bill didn't seem to struggle with the ins and outs, why and why nots of any decision to try something new and live with any uncertainty that might exist. The "why not" for Bill is a giving in to what that experience might offer in terms of meeting new people, living in a new location, and the excitement of the challenge to succeed. Similarly, Bill began to view his journey of stroke recovery as an opportunity to learn, to grow, to be challenged, and to meet new people along the way.

REFERENCE

Laal, M., & Salamati, P. (2012). Life-long learning; Why do we need it? *Procedia-Social and Behavioral Sciences, 31*, 399–403. Retrieved from https://www.sciencedirect.com/science/article/pii/S1877042811030023

---

1. Life-Long Learning (LLL) is the continuous building of skills and knowledge throughout the life of an individual. It not only enhances social inclusion, active citizenship and personal development, but also competitiveness and employability (p. 399) (Laal & Salamati, 2012).

PART 2

COMMUNICATION LESSONS LEARNED

The chapters in Part Two solidify and expand the lessons we learned in Part One, helping us to recognize the ways in which communication practices cultivate resilience in the midst of health crises. We learn that a key component of resilience is believing in your own abilities and communicating those with others. We also learn that some of us are better than others at communicating what we need and that our competencies in communicating are essential to good health outcomes. Finally, we learn that we all need a good support system to sustain our recovery—we can't do it alone.

The first lesson about communication to take to heart is the critical role that self-efficacy plays in our recovery. Self-efficacy is an individual's perception that they have the ability to achieve an outcome through their own actions (Bandura, 1977, 1986, 1997; Lee, Arthur, & Avis, 2008). People with high self-efficacy tend to keep trying at something even when they fail, especially when they receive encouragement from others to keep trying (Brouwer-Goossensen et al., 2018). Bill began to develop a stronger sense of self-efficacy when he agreed to be seen in public to have lunch with Debbie Moore, an occupational therapist at Sharp Hospital. It was just 2 weeks after his stroke and Bill was still in the hospital and really didn't want to be seen by anyone. It was a critical moment when he recognized how important it was for him to continue to take steps like this if he was going to progress in his recovery. Actor Kirk Douglas served as a role model for Bill; he saw that Douglas did not allow ableist views to keep him from speaking with his aphasia in front of an audience of millions. Witnessing Douglas's speech encouraged Bill to take his recovery into his own hands; he proclaimed, "if he can do it, I can do it." This moment became the inspiration for Bill's critical first step toward facing his discomfort in being disabled. It allowed him to place himself in public situations that would give him opportunities to practice speech and movement. For instance, Bill began to take himself on trips to the local mall, going up and down escalators and into and out of stores as he practiced moving with a cane.

In his life before the stroke, Bill learned to how to build a strong sense of self-efficacy, even in situations where he was placed at a disadvantage. For instance, on the racquetball court, Bill could never expect to go head-to-head with champion-level friends who had more natural speed and strength than he did. Yet, rather than becoming frustrated and giving up, Bill trusted in his own ability to find alternative ways to best his opponents. As Charlie told us, "[Bill] didn't try to do something with what he didn't have. He tried to do something with what he did have. And he persisted in it without complaint and without a negative attitude …. He developed his own game, where he was maybe the top amateur of the club." The same friends who encouraged him to keep playing racquetball before the stroke encouraged him to hang out, have lunch, and keep striving to improve, contributing to Bill's motivation and belief in his own ability to recover. For instance, Tom reported that he "would make sure that Billy had access to plain, solid research that supported the idea that your mind is part of your body … and re-confirmed his beliefs that he could heal." These supportive messages from friends helped Bill to develop and maintain a strong sense of self-efficacy even during the most difficult phases of his recovery.

The second lesson about communication that can be drawn from the chapters in Part Two, and throughout the whole book, is the critical importance of our social networks and strong ties with the people in our network (Abbott, 2014; Mattson & Hall, 2011). Research reveals that constructing positive relationships with family, friends, and health care professionals is one of the best predictors of a high-quality life (Nussbaum 2017; Nussbaum, Robinson, & Grew, 1985). Strong ties in these relationships often translate to an abundance of social support when we face health crises, such as the one that Bill faced (Mattson & Hall, 2011). Bill has a knack for creating strong ties with people who have become lifelong friends. Dr. Bud tells us that the group of racquetball players maintained their strong friendship with Bill after his stroke. He reports that Bill "was always included, he was always there, so we were basically a support group. We didn't even notice the affliction, but we kept praising him for his recovery. He has to take the credit for being so persistent, but we wouldn't let him quit either."

In the language of social network analysis, Bill has developed a dense network of strong social ties. As a result, he had access to a built-in "support group" during his stroke recovery process. This group provided instrumental support[1] by driving him to appointments (Sheila), providing extra therapy (Phil), and taking him for wheelchair laps around the hospital (Charlie). Additionally, friends like Tom provided appraisal, esteem, and informational support. Tom describes how he assisted Bill framing stroke recovery as a mind-over-matter process of healing oneself. In doing so, he nurtured Bill's sense of self-efficacy. As the prototypical professor, Tom reinforced this appraisal support with "access to plain, solid research"—informational support corroborating the idea that "your mind is part of your body."

---

1. Typically, social support is classified into five types: "*informational support* (e.g., giving advice or sharing information) *instrumental support* (e.g., assisting with tasks or providing resources), *appraisal support* (e.g., offering new perspectives), *esteem support* (e.g., enhancing self-worth and feelings about abilities, attributes, or accomplishments), and *emotional support* (e.g., expressing care, empathy, and acceptance) (Yamasaki, 2017).

Beyond providing instrumental, appraisal, and informational support, however, Bill's network of friends served as a repository of shared experiences. In fact, Sheila notes that her main approach to supporting Bill post-stroke was to simply make sure that he "remembered stuff from a long time ago." "Talking about old stuff" served a practical purpose in that it tested Bill's cognitive abilities post-stroke. More than this, the practice of reminiscing with old friends grounded Bill in joyful memories, feeding his will to survive and thrive during a time when he was tempted to give in to depression and despair.

Repeatedly, Bill's friends talked about not treating Bill any differently after his stroke. Instead, they described simply accepting his new physical challenges and unpredictable emotions (esteem and emotional support). Bill's friends sought to create spaces in which he might feel less vulnerable and more willing to take a risk. Even now, when Bill has nearly fully recovered from his stroke, Charlie talks about using own health challenges as a tool to make Bill feel "a little safer" in potentially identity-threatening situations, such as returning to the racquetball court. Our conversation with Charlie illustrates a key dialectical tension between "accepting in the midst" and "pushing the putt." Charlie recognizes that accepting his friend—slobber and all—also means helping Bill to confront his own excuses. While others may continue to praise Bill for his recovery successes, Charlie acknowledges his friend's lingering sadness, challenging him to "stretch." While the ties that link Bill's social network are strong, they are also bidirectional.[2] His relationships are defined by a sense of reciprocal support and mutual obligation. Our interviewees explained how they helped Bill throughout his recovery process, yet their responses were also characterized by a profound sense of gratitude for all of the ways in which Bill's friendship had enriched their lives.

A third related lesson that can be drawn from the stories in Part Two relates to communication competence generally (Cupach, Canary, & Spitzberg, 2010; Hannawa & Spitzberg, 2015) but specifically to forms of communication that are central to communication competence (Spitzberg, 2013).[3] Attentiveness is a competence where a person's style of communication shows attention to, interest in, and concern for another (e.g., listening, displaying empathy, and asking questions) (Spitzberg, 2013). Clearly, Joy, Clee, and all of Bill's friends were attentive to his needs, helping him to practice new skills—Joy in training Bill, Clee in assisting Bill in connecting things that were not connected, Dr. Bud in praising Bill when he noticed progress in his recovery, and Tom in sitting with Bill in the hospital. Tom's attentiveness in displaying empathy is clear when he states "I stayed with him for quite a while … He was crying, and I was holding his hand and telling him it was going to be okay." While these are communication skills essential for health care providers to enact with patients, we can see how Bill and his supportive friends utilized these skills in their interactions throughout his recovery.

2. Social network analysis explores the ways that our ties with others can be weak or strong depending on our patterns of interaction with one another and the kinds of conversations we engage in with the people in our networks. While it is most beneficial to have some strong ties, often people with a large number of weak ties can gain healthy benefits as well (Jones, Ferreday, & Hodgson, 2008).
3. Spitzberg (2013) discusses four communication competencies essential for health care providers, including attentiveness, composure, coordination, and expressiveness.

Undoubtedly, most of these lessons in communication are linked to positive health outcomes (Street, Makoul, Arora, & Epstein, 2009). However, it isn't always easy for stroke survivors and their support network to communicate through the inevitable dialectic tensions they experience in their relationships. Research has revealed that the ability of people stroke survivor relationships to communicate about dialectic tensions, such as uncertainty–acceptance, realism–idealism, and self-orientation–partner orientation, can open lines of communication and improve people's health and their relationships (Brann, Himes, Dillow, & Weber, 2010).[4]

REFERENCES

Abbott, K. (2014). Social networks: Overall. In T. L. Thompson (Ed.), *Encyclopedia of health communication* (pp. 1302–1305). Los Angeles, CA: Sage.

Bandura, A. (1977). Self-efficacy: Toward a unifying theory of behavioral change. *Psychological Review, 84*, 191–215.

Bandura, A. (1986). *Social foundations of thought and action: A social cognitive theory*. Englewood Cliffs, NJ: Prentice-Hall.

Bandura, A. (1997). Self-Efficacy: *The exercise of control*. New York, NY: W. H. Freeman.

Brann, M., Himes, K. L., Dillow, M. R., & Weber, K. (2010). Dialectic tensions in stroke survivor relationships. *Health Communication, 25*, 323–332.

Brouwer-Goossensen, D., van Genugten, L., Lingsma, H. F., Dippel, D. W. J., Koudstaal, P. J., & den Hertog, H. M. (2018). Self-efficacy for health-related behavior change in patients with TIA or minor ischemic stroke. *Psychology & Health, 33*, 1490–1501. https://doi.org/10.1080/08870446.2018.1508686

Cupach, W. R., Canary, D. J., & Spitzberg, B. H. (2010). *Competence in interpersonal conflict* (2nd ed.). Long Grove, IL: Waveland.

Hannawa, A. F., & Spitzberg, B. H. (Eds.). (2015). *Communication competence*. Boston, MA: De Gruyter.

Jones, C. R., Ferreday, D., & Hodgson, V. (2008). Networked learning a relational approach: Weak and strong ties. *Journal of Computer Assisted Learning, 24*, 90–102.

Lee, L. L., Arthur, A., & Avis, M. (2008). Using self-efficacy theory to develop interventions that help older people overcome psychological barriers to physical activity: A discussion paper. *International Journal of Nursing Studies, 45*, 1690–1699. doi:10.1016/j.ijnurstu.2008.02.012

Mattson, M., & Hall, J. G. (2011). *Health communication as nexus: A service-learning approach*. Dubuque, IA: Kendall Hunt.

---

4. According the Brann et al. (2010), the uncertainty–acceptance dialectic relates to the tension between uncertainty regarding the future and the possibility of another stroke and the acceptance related to the thankfulness and appreciation that the person is still alive. The realism–idealism dialectic relates to the tension between the reality of the present situation, including frustration and sorrow, and the idealistic and optimistic views of recovery. The self-orientation–partner orientation dialectic relates to tensions between the needs and preferences of the stroke survivor and of the partner caring for them.

Nussbaum, J. F. (2017). Quality communication across the life span. In J. Yamasaki, P. Geist-Martin, & B. F. Sharf (Eds.), *Storied health communication: Communicating personal, cultural, and political complexities* (pp. 161–162). Long Gove, IL: Waveland.

Nussbaum, J. F., Robinson, J. D., & Grew, D. J. (1985). Communication behavior of the long-term health care employee: Implications for the elderly resident. *Communication Research Reports, 2*, 1622.

Street, R. L., Jr., Makoul, G., Arora, N. K., & Epstein, R. M. (2009). How does communication heal? Pathways linking clinician–patient communication to health outcomes. *Patient Education and Counseling, 74*, 295–301.

Spitzberg, B. H. (2013). (Re)Introducing communication competence to the health professions. *Journal of Public Health Research, 2*, 126–135.

Yamasaki, J. (2017). Communicating health and connection in supportive communities. In J. Yamasaki, P. Geist-Martin, & B. F. Sharf (Eds.), *Storied health and illness: Communicating personal, cultural, and political complexities* (pp. 251–271). Long Grove, IL: Waveland.

PART 3

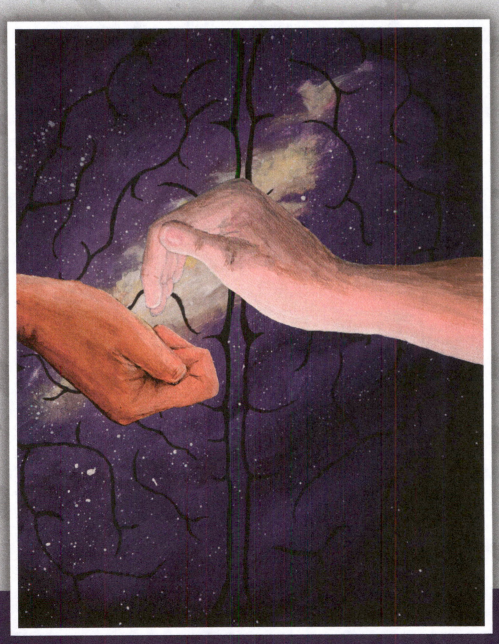

"The wounded storyteller is anyone who has suffered and lived to tell the tale. Suffering does not magically disappear when the tale is told, but the more stories I heard the less space my own suffering seemed to take." (p. vi)
—Arthur W. Frank, *The Wounded Storyteller: Body, Illness, & Ethics, 2nd ed.*

"As wounded, people may be cared for, but as storytellers, they care for others. The ill, and those who suffer, can also be healers. Their injuries become the source of the potency of their stories …. Because stories can heal, the wounded healer and the wounded storyteller are not separate, but different aspects of the same figure …. Seriously ill people are wounded not just in body but in voice. They need to become storytellers in order to recover the voice that illness and its treatment often take away." (p. xx)
—Arthur W. Frank, *The Wounded Storyteller: Body, Illness, & Ethics, 2nd ed.*

Moving from *Part Two* to *Part Three*, we see the expansion of Bill's passion for sharing his story with other stroke survivors. He takes advantage of every opportunity to tell people what he has learned about falling in love with the process of his recovery. In Chapters 12 and 13 we learn the steps that Bill has taken to "pay it forward" and help other stroke survivors. Bill's story becomes preventative medicine, helping raise awareness about stroke in a culture where many people are unaware of stroke's signs and symptoms. We also learn how others—including friends, professors, providers, and students—value the work he has accomplished as a stroke advocate. In Chapter 14, we explore the emotional challenges that Bill has faced in doing his advocacy work; he experiences frustration and disappointment when the people he has attempted to help do not call back and do not persist in their process of recovery. In our closing chapter, Chapter 15, we take a close look at the ways that Bill has been recognized for his advocacy work, considering how programs like Sharp Hospital's Victories of Spirit can provide the positive reinforcement that peer mentors like Bill need in order to continue their work as advocates.

CHAPTER 12

"You Sincerely Care about What Happens to Other People": From Salesman to Advocate

We sit side-by-side on the soft, white leather couches in Patricia's front room, surrounded by stacks of yellow file folders. They contain the accumulated evidence of Bill's dynamic life—news clippings, hospital brochures, typed student feedback on Bill's many visits to Patricia's Health Communication class, photographs, and Bill's personal accounts, typed in his preferred blue Calibri font. Papers scatter across the coffee table like fallen leaves, the physical remnants of experiences from seasons passed.

Sarah sighs audibly, exhaling through a sudden wave of anxiety. "There's so much here!" she says, turning to Patricia in search of guidance.

"I know," Patricia responds, sounding similarly overwhelmed. "It's difficult to know where to start." We sift through folders together, squinting at random papers like a pair of fortunetellers trying to read tea leaves. "Look at this," Patricia murmurs after a few minutes, handing Sarah a single yellowed sheet of paper filled with blocky, typewriter-style letters. It is a note written over 30 years ago by Dr. Tom Gillette, Bill's former professor and close friend, giving Bill feedback on his communication style at the peak of his career as a salesman. Sarah reads over Patricia's shoulder, smiling as she remembers Tom's warm, richly resonant voice.

Patricia looks at Sarah with a meaningfully raised eyebrow as she reads the final snippet of Tom's note aloud: "No wonder you are a great sales person. You would also be a great therapist. Come to think of it, I believe you are." Tom's words sound like the prophecy we have been searching for. They sum up the link between Bill's earlier lives as a teacher and a salesman and his present life as a stroke advocate, illustrating the ways in which he adapted the communication skills he had honed in these professions to his new calling as a mentor.

> Another wonderful things about you, you don't make major mistakes in communication. What don't you do?
>
> You do not order, direct, or command. That communicates unacceptance and may produce fear and resentment.
>
> You do not admonish or threaten. That makes people fearful, submissive, and eventually evokes hostility.
>
> You do not preach or moralize. That suggests you don't have confidence in the other person (when you do it) and may arouse resistance and even guilt.
>
> You don't lecture or teach, though you do provide adequate data. This means you don't put the other person in a one-down situation, though you do encourage colleagueship.
>
> - Finally, though this is only partial, you are not a phony. You are real when you are with someone and they sense and know that. No one really likes a phony. They might stick around in the beginning, but it is temporary at best.
>
> And I suppose I should mention that you are personal rather than impersonal, informal rather than formal, and that you sincerely care about what happens to people. No wonder you are a great sales person. You would also be a great therapist. Come to bink of it, I believe you are.
>
> So good luck on the seminar-----...

Tom

In his short note, Tom manages to summarize some of the key aspects of Bill's communication style that have been so evident in our interaction with him and in the stories that others have told us about him. Bill manages to connect so well with others because he cultivates "colleagueship," constantly communicating his belief in the basic goodness and competence of those he encounters. As Tom notes, people respond to Bill's genuine interest in their well-being. He writes,

> You [Bill] are not a phony. You are real when you are with someone and they sense and know that. No one really likes a phony. They might stick around in the beginning, but it is temporary at best …. You sincerely care about what happens to people.

This last assertion from Tom—that Bill sincerely cares about what happens to people—is the main thrust of Bill's commitment to becoming a stroke advocate. Bill's friend, the racquetball champion, Charlie Brumfield, voiced a similar link between Bill's approach to stroke advocacy and his former life as a teacher. "When you're teaching … you have to develop a patience and a persistence and really love. You have to convey your love to the other people or they can't learn," he explained to us. "They'll wiggle out of the learning process and rebel against authority. So, part of it is you've gotta communicate the love to them, but you also have to provide a general push. And he is an expert of doing that." Bill tells us that, in the midst of his recovery, he "made a promise to [him]self that if [he] got better, [he] would become an advocate for stroke survivors." Debbie Moore, a recreation therapist at Sharp Hospital, told us that she had seen similar sentiments inspire other patients to return as advocates. "I think they get that feeling right when they're here as an inpatient," she explained, "They're not ready yet to [advocate], but they're like, 'I want to come back and volunteer here.' They just want to be a part of the recovery of other people and give back some."

In this chapter, we explore how Bill worked with local hospitals to connect with fellow stroke survivors and reveal the valuable role that peer mentors like Bill play in supporting patients' recovery. We draw on interviews with several of the health care providers and administrators who witnessed Bill's advocacy work, and who are responsible for developing and coordinating peer mentor programs in rehabilitation facilities. Along the way, we'll share several examples of Bill's success stories.

FACING THE CONSTRAINTS OF THE U.S. HEALTH CARE SYSTEM

Health care providers and administrators who we spoke with repeated a refrain of frustration with the constraints that insurance companies placed on patients' access to long-term, acute rehabilitation services. Bill faced many of these constraints in the challenging months of recovery after his stroke. They also weighed heavily on Bill in his role as a stroke advocate after his recovery. For instance, we spoke with Dan Hanzlik, Manager of Business Development for Sharp Rehab, who manages a team of eight nurses who go out into the community and assess patients to see if they're eligible for inpatient acute rehabilitation. Dan described the tightrope patients walk as they attempt to retain access to care while also making progress in their recovery. "[Patients] have to be sick enough so that they need to be there, but they can't be too well [so] that they don't need to be there." He noted that the criteria for who merits acute rehab continue to become more and more narrow, meaning that fewer people have access acute rehab. Dan elaborated,

> It's all about cost-benefit [analysis] …. All care in the United States is being pushed down to lower levels of care. And it's happening with us as well. There are far more people who even five years ago would have been appropriate for acute rehab, they now go to skilled nursing facilities, which is less intensive, less structured, less physician involvement, less nursing involvement. And I expect that you'll see more and more and more of that. It will not change …. We used to take patients 20 years ago for an average of 30 days, 35 days. The average they stay now in San Diego is about 12-13 days. I don't think they are getting better any faster. A lot of that [care] is going onto those people at home—those wives and family members and husbands.

Interview contributed by Debbie Moore. Copyright © Kendall Hunt Publishing Company.

Recreation therapist, Debbie Moore, noted that these systemic constraints often force health care providers to focus on helping people to simply be able to accomplish the basic functions of daily living—like buttoning a shirt or showering—on their own, or with minimal assistance from others. These low bars for recovery serve insurance companies' desire to get patients "out the door" as quickly as possible.

It is incredibly challenging to provide patients with the kind of therapy they need to recover within the tiny time windows prescribed by insurance agencies. Stephanie Ousley, a recreation therapist at Grossmont hospital, noted that, while insurance agencies sometimes covered longer stays in a nursing home, such facilities tend to offer fewer specialized therapies less often—perhaps three times a week. Meanwhile, Stephanie noted, patients who were released home or who went to a nursing home frequently struggled with depression and other psychosocial challenges related to adjusting to life post-stroke. She explained,

> For Bill, [the stroke] financially devastated him and wiped him out. [Stroke] does that for a lot of people. The statistics are showing that strokes are happening at a younger and younger age ... now if we're seeing more and more strokes in the 40s and 50s, what does that do? Maybe you're the primary breadwinner .... Maybe you may lose your home. People lose everything because they have to get down to now where they're a part of the Medi-Cal or Medicaid system. You can't have any money then [because making too much would disqualify you from collecting disability benefits]. So, you're kind of stuck. It's like, "Oh gosh, now I've lost everything." You're dependent upon the system for everything .... It's like, "Oh my gosh, how do you ride the bus when you've had a disability?"

Stephanie's comments outline a system of care that fails not only to address patients' physical needs but also their needs related to finances, transportation, and mental health/identity.

However, the providers we talked to were not without hope. Primarily, their hope was tied to outpatient and community programming. Debbie Moore emphasized that resources have proliferated across the 36 years of her career, creating a dense network of educational, recreational, and advocacy-related resources beyond specific treatment programs. As a recreational therapist, Debbie has played a significant role in developing such resources. Her work focuses on helping stroke survivors to (re)gain the ability to participate in activities that not only address their wide-ranging needs but give them a sense of joy and normalcy. When we sat down with Debbie, she gave us an overview of the recreational therapy program at Sharp. "What we want to do is rehabilitate the whole person," she explained,

> You don't want to get a person walking or using their wheelchair and then [forget] about the rest of their life. We feel like we help get people back to doing quality, productive leisure lifestyles. Things that they enjoy. We start out, we ask them, what is it you like to do in your

Interview contributed by Stephanie Ousley. Copyright © Kendall Hunt Publishing Company.

FALLING IN LOVE WITH THE PROCESS: CULTIVATING RESILIENCE IN HEALTH CRISES

free time? … We ask them what they like to do, and then based on that, then we develop a treatment plan. What we try to do is, we do what we call leisure education, where we educate them about adaptive leisure. For example, the paraplegic might not know that he could go adapted snow skiing again, or adapted water skiing …. It's based on a philosophy of leisure and that value and that self-efficacy, leisure efficacy. You're doing what you enjoy and we would like to help people keep that as they adjust to the semi-disabled or partially disabled …. We do inpatient [recreational therapy], but then we also have a community program. We hook them up with our newsletter and then we plan adaptive sports, fitness, recreation. We have ongoing programs and we have seasonal programs.

SHARP COMMUNITY PROGRAMS

SPORTS, RECREATION, AND WELLNESS PROGRAMS

Sharp Rehabilitation Sports, Recreation and Wellness Program is known for integrating physically challenged individuals into the community. These programs are open to anyone with a physical disability and are offered at Sharp Rehabilitation Center, Sharp Grossmont Rehabilitation Center, Sharp Coronado. Please call for enrollment information.

SHARP MEMORIAL REHAB CENTER	SHARP GROSSMONT REHAB CENTER	SHARP CORONADO HOSPITAL
Adaptive Weight Training & Fitness Class Mondays & Wednesdays 4:30-6:0 pm $25.00 for 3 month session 858-939-3048 debra.moore@sharp.com	**Adaptive Aquatics** Mondays, Wednesdays, Thursdays, Fridays $60.00 once/week for 8 weeks	**Gentle Fitness** Tuesday and Thursday 10:00-11:00 am **Qi Gong, Yoga, Fitness, and Tai Chi Classes**
Adaptive Yoga Mondays, 4:00-5:00pm $30.00 for 6 weeks or $7.00 per class 800-827-4277 www.sharp.com/health-classes/ adaptive-yoga-class-1708	**Arthritis Aquatic Program** Monday thru Saturday 7:00am-7:00pm $104.00 for 8 weeks-2xweek $156.00 for 8 weeks-3x per week **Aquacise** Tuesdays and Thursdays, 8:55-9:50am $104.00 for 8 wk session-2x/week	**For Coronado Programs,** **619-522-3798** nicole.dangelo@sharp.com http://www.sharp.com/ hospitals/coronado/sewall- healthy-living-center/ calendar.cfm? utm_source=Print&utm_mediu m=Vanity&utm_campaign=hlc
Adaptive Golf Clinic Thursdays, 3:00-4:00pm 858-939-3048 bernadette.gore@sharp.com	**AiChi** Tuesdays and Thursdays 7:10pm $104.00 for 8 wk session-2x/wk	
Gentle Fitness Thursdays 1:00-2:00pm $30.00 for 6 weeks, or $5.00 / class 858-939-3048 wendy.pierce@sharp.com	**SPLASH₂O - Special Kids Learn Aquatic Skills in H₂O** Mondays, Wednesdays and Saturdays, 10:15am $60.00 for 8 week session	
SEASONAL EVENTS • Ski Trip • Sharp Quad Rugby • Day on the Bay • Adaptive Sailing • Adaptive Surfing	**Adaptive Golf Clinic** Saturdays, 9:30-10:30am 619-740-4104 **Gentle Fitness** Tuesday 9:30-10:30am $88.00 for 8 weeks-twice/wk 619-740-4104 grace.latimer@sharp.com	**STROKE CLUBS** **YESS (Young Enthusiastic Stroke Survivors)** Days and Times vary 858-939-3048 bernadette.gore@sharp.com **Communication Group** **Speech Therapy Dept.** Thursdays 1:45-2:45 pm $35.00 per month 619-740-6055 marissa.pabis@sharp.com
For Memorial Programs, **858-939-3048**	**For Grossmont Programs,** **619-740-4104** elizabeth.clarno@sharp.com	

For more information about Sharp Rehab Recreation Therapy
http://www.sharp.com/search/?q=recreation+therapy

From Sharp HealthCare. Reprinted by permission.

Examples of community programming at Sharp

Debbie's description of the recreation therapy program captures an ethos of well-being and holistic health that has begun to shape health care in the United States, supporting an integrative approach that seeks to address patients' psychosocial needs alongside their physical ones.

Dan Hanzlik noted that some of the most effective recreational therapy programming at Sharp was developed, at least in part, by patients themselves. For instance, two former patients were inspired by their shared love of lacrosse to create an adaptive lacrosse program, expanding this community resource to over 30 clinics. This example highlights the vital role that peer advocates, like Bill, play in the "recovery community."

BECOMING A PEER MENTOR

Our interviewees highlighted several ways in which peer mentors were incorporated in programming for stroke survivors. Sharp and Grossmont hospitals both have official peer mentor programs, connecting current patients with positive stroke survivor role models who might be better equipped to empathize, educate, and motivate. While Bill's role as a peer mentor was comparably a fairly informal one,[1] much of the work that he accomplished fits with the kinds of goals that the hospitals' formal programs were designed to achieve.

Stephanie at Grossmont Hospital described a highly structured peer visitor program, where volunteers attend weekly meetings to review specific patient cases, keep updated on the latest stroke research, and brainstorm new strategies to connect with patients. Peer visitors at Grossmont also engage in educational outreach, attending health fairs and other local events to teach the public how to prevent, recognize, and respond to stroke. Beyond the official peer visitors program, however, Stephanie noted the important work that stroke advocates accomplished in the everyday, spontaneous encounters with strangers. "No matter where they're at—they could be at church, they could be playing Bingo, they could be seeing somebody on the bus—they're always advocating," she explained. "All of our peer visitors do that. They'll look and they'll go, 'That person will typically have a stroke.' They'll strike up a conversation with them."

Dan Hanzlik explained the nature of Sharp Hospital's ambassador program, where volunteers come in to talk with people who have recently experienced a stroke. Bill participated in Sharp's ambassador program for a decade. "Bill has been doing this for us now for close to ten years," Dan noted, adding, "Bill had a challenging stay here. I didn't round[2] on him. I wasn't one of his rounders, but my understanding was that he really struggled when he first got here. It was hard for him to gain some momentum in his own therapy, but you know he has that positive attitude; he is never a quit guy."

---

1. Sharp has since tightened some of the policies associated with their peer mentor program, making it more difficult for Bill to simply drop by or to receive calls from nurses about a particular patient.
2. Slang for participating in patient rounds, where a health care team observes the patient and goes over the specifics of their case

In his time visiting Sharp, Bill built a rapport with therapists and other providers who recognized his passion for stroke advocacy. Debbie Moore recalled picking up the phone to call Bill when she recognized a patient's need for peer support. "There is this woman, this patient I'm seeing, and she's really having a hard time," she'd say, "I think it would be really good for you to come in and talk to her, encourage her. She's not very hopeful. She doesn't want to come out and do the [recreational therapy] groups. I really want you to see her, encourage her." Many of Bill's most touching stories of stroke advocacy stem from interactions that began in this way—including this story of his encounter with a young mother.

STROKE ADVOCACY STORY: MARCELLA

"First of all, strokes don't discriminate by age," Bill emphasizes. "They happen in the fetus all the way up, but it's just more likely in older people because of blood pressure and cholesterol and all that."

"This young lady at Sharp, she was 28. The staff called me, and I went to see her. She had an ischemic stroke on the left side, like mine. Her biggest worry was taking care of her new baby. I said, 'One of things that you can do, you can still hold the baby with your left hand. You hold it against you, so that the baby can hear your heartbeat, feel your heartbeat. Then you can exercise your arm by trying to bring it up to the baby.' I showed her a few more exercises, but that was the main one. I felt it was so important. I said, 'You're going to be fine. Don't worry about your leg right now. What you do is, at night, hold your leg. Just listen to the music. Tap your foot. It won't tap, but just keep tapping. Think about it. Do you have a rocking chair? Take your baby, rock with the baby, sing to the baby. Rock, rock, rock and do that for 15 minutes, 10 minutes, 5 minutes, and you're going to get better, and we will both cry.'

"I saw her a month later. They called me up and said, 'She is up here and wants to see you.' So, I went up to see her. She says, 'Thank you, Mr. Torres.'

I said, 'No, no. We are both in the same position. We both had a stroke, so we have to support each other. The most important thing is the baby.'

She says, 'Watch.' She brought her hand up. She says, 'I can't hold her, but I can bring my arm up and touch her.' I cried a flood of tears!

I haven't heard from her since then. Usually, I don't hear from them. They go on with their own life, but I always say, 'Here's my number. Call me.'"

Interview contributed by Daniel Hanzlik. Copyright © Kendall Hunt Publishing Company.

Bill's stories of his advocacy with stroke survivors like Marcella reveal the depth of his passion for this work, but also his impact on patients. But we wanted to know more. So, we set up a meeting with David Brown, the System Director of Sharp Healthcare Rehabilitation Services and someone who is familiar with Bill both as a former patient and a stroke advocate.

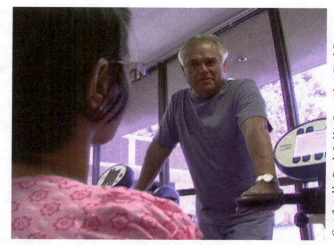

Bill working with a stroke survivor

***

"We really appreciate you taking the time to meet with us," Sarah says, seating herself at the mahogany-colored desk in David Brown's office as they wait for Patricia to park the car. Sarah is suddenly self-conscious, recognizing that David likely has more pressing tasks to accomplish than speaking with two researchers about a former patient.

"You're very welcome," David responds graciously, "Bill's a great guy."

"He is a pretty good guy," Sarah agrees, just as Patricia knocks on the open office door.

"Hi there! Sorry to be a little late," she says, sounding breathless.

"That's alright. I heard you were having a parking issue," David says, offering Patricia a seat. "We just put a new parking process in place about six weeks ago," he adds with an apologetic smile, "There are a few little bit bumps."

As Patricia settles into her chair, David returns to his description of Bill. "He's really an amazing guy for what he has done with his life and giving back to people. I just don't know a lot of people who do that."

"That's what we are interested in understanding," Sarah says. "What makes a person like Bill so effective as stroke advocate and peer mentor?"

"I've talked to people about the influence that he's had in their lives." David leans back in his office chair, reflecting. "He's really turned people's minds around. I think the most compelling thing when I think about him is, he's so damn positive. I think it's difficult with strokes because you don't really know what you're going to get or what you're not going to get. Bill tells stroke survivors, 'You have to be patient about the whole thing. Just keep on working at it.'"

"I think the power of Bill is that he doesn't forget. He remembers his experience. He remembers what he went through, he remembers the hard work. He remembers being frustrated and being angry about everything. He really works exceptionally well with stroke patients because he's got that background and that history behind him, and he knows exactly what they are going through because he went through it himself."

"He is always there," David enthuses, leaning forward on his desk. "He always makes himself available to patients. If they run into a problem even after they get home, I know that he gives them his number to be able to give him a call. He'll come out and see them at their home. He really is the full package."

David pauses, looking thoughtful. "I think he has said this to me in the past—he probably would not be the person he is right now unless he went through what he went through," he explains. "He is so grateful for what he has and the recovery that he has made, and he's so grateful for the fact that he can give back at the same time. It has become a part of his being—it truly has become a part of his being, to give back and to help people."

"Have you seen some of his work, first hand?" Sarah asks.

"He drops in and shows it to me," David says, smiling at memories of Bill's success stories. "He came in last week and told me about an individual that he was working with. The individual had a stroke years ago and their hand was clenched. He would work with him to open up the hand and he brought me the picture of the individual's hand being opened. He was so proud of it. That is no small feat by any means, because it is painful—it's really painful and uncomfortable after that amount of time. But you know what? He is diligent. He just doesn't give up. He's like a dog with a bone on him."

Sarah and Patricia nod their heads listening intently to David's characterization of Bill, confirming that this is the Bill they know so well.

"He does work with aphasia patients also," David continues. "He'll play around to find out where he can get to so that he perceives that the patient can understand what's going on, what's happening. That is no small task by any means. But he is intuitive, because he has been there and he knows the frustrations he had. Like I said, he has learned so much from his past experiences. He uses those when he ends up working with other patients."

"OK, so he's calling from his experiences and testing it out in his work with stroke survivors," Sarah paraphrases. "Do they respond to this or to that?"

David nods. "What may work with one patient may not work with another patient. Like I said, he's intuitive, and it's a trial-and-error process. You know Bill," David adds. "Bill will touch—he's not a distance away. He'll hold your hand, he'll put his hand on your arm, which honestly in many ways is very therapeutic. There's a lot of people—even families and loved ones—who are scared. They don't know what to do or what not to do. They stand back, and Bill is like right in there." As he describes this characteristic of Bill, David holds his hands together in front of him, just a few inches apart, illustrating the close physical proximity that Bill maintains with patients. "He touches you, which brings a level of comfort," he explains. "It brings a level of warmth into the whole experience."

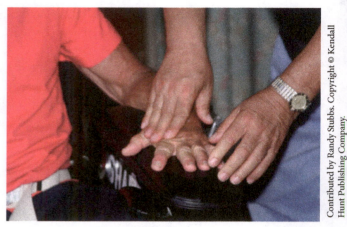

Bill working with a stroke survivor

"That's interesting to think about," Sarah replies, "Part of our field in health communication includes studying nonverbal communication and how factors like touch shape relationships in healthcare settings."

"He talks directly to the person," David expands, recognizing that eye contact is an equally important aspect of nonverbal communication. "I've seen situations where there are family members there and, for some reason, we the providers don't talk to the patient—we talk to the family members. Bill talks directly to the patient because the patient is the focus. The patient is the most important thing there, and he recognizes that."

"He told us a story about singing happy birthday with the patient; he said that you were there," Patricia says.

"Yes," David smiles, "He was singing happy birthday to Rose."

STROKE ADVOCACY STORY: ROSE

"What can I say about Rose?" Bill reminisces, "A rose by any other name cannot compare to this Rose."

"One afternoon I was visiting recreational rehab at Sharp Hospital. One of the therapists approached me and told me about a wonderful and beautiful woman by the name of Rose in the stroke ward. She was depressed and just giving up. The therapist asked if I would talk to her. Of course, I said yes. But first I asked her if she would speak to Rose and give her my background. She went in and explained to Rose that I had spent over a month in the same room. I was given permission and in I went. What a surprise! Not only was she beautiful, but she also looked like royalty. But she was depressed she had aphasia and hadn't spoken a word in a week. The conversation went like this: 'Rose, my name is Bill and I had a stroke just like yours. Mine was on the left side and I couldn't speak either.' She looked at me with her beautiful, soulful eyes. She tried to smile."

"I knew her stroke was on the left side of the brain which affects speech. However, the right side of the brain is the music side. I asked Rose if she would do me a big favor. I said, 'Rose, today is my birthday. Could you all sing Happy Birthday to me?' She looked at me as if I were nuts, but she shook her head yes. I said on the count of three we'll begin. One, two, three …. Happy Birthday to you … and she started singing and had a beautiful voice."

"The therapists and I started crying, but Rose kept on singing. Oh, what joy! We hugged and I said from now on she could start singing for her supper. Her eyes were all lit up and a wonderful smile was evident. Wow, that felt good. To quote a line from a Cole Porter song, 'What moments divine, what rapture serene.'"

"The next day I went back to the hospital. I was unaware that news of what happened the day before had spread. When I entered, the Head of Rehab came out of his office and gave me a big hug with tears in his eyes. He called out, 'Bill's here!' People came out of their offices and started applauding. I was speechless. What a feeling! There weren't words that could express my thanks."

***

"It was so enlightening and enriching and moving for the patients." David remembers, "Bill, in many ways, has become a clinician. He's learned all of these little different things that work that you wouldn't think would normally work at all. Like I said, he's a joy, and he's a such a resource and incredibly valuable asset to us."

While Bill's initial attempts to "give back" frequently involve kind of one-on-one peer mentorship encounters described above, Bill also became a frequent speaker for organizations related to stroke and brain injury recovery.

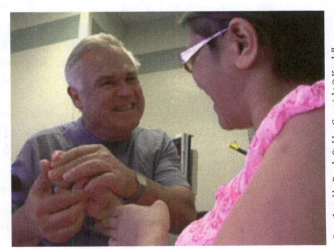

Bill working with a stroke survivor

BECOMING A MOTIVATIONAL SPEAKER

What we learn from so many of Bill's stories is that as David said, "he is never a quit guy," always looking for new opportunities to be an advocate for stroke survivors. His speaking engagements produced several meaningful encounters with stroke survivors, including this one with Delray.

Stroke Advocacy Story: Delray

"One day I was going to give a talk at a Stroke Survivors meeting at the VA Hospital," Bill recounts. "Before the meeting, I was speaking to one of the therapists that had helped me. She pointed to Delray, who was in the office. She said she was trying to get him to walk, but he wouldn't even try. Delray was a stroke survivor who was in a wheelchair and didn't look too happy. The therapist asked me if I would talk to him. I said yes and went over to him. The therapist had told me that Delray had been in therapy over a year and was very depressed and would not try to walk for fear of falling."

"After the introductions, I asked him why he was depressed. He said he was tired of being in a wheelchair. I asked him if he had tried to walk. He said he was afraid he'd fall. Speaking from experience, I knew the feeling. From a sitting position one must get up and actually start a falling process and then stand. That little bit of letting gravity pull you toward the floor is somewhat scary. Normally, we just do it and don't think about it."

"I shared my story of getting out of a wheelchair and how frightened I was, and we laughed about it. With his permission, I checked his legs for strength and flexibility. I said 'Delray, how would you like to walk into the meeting? Would you give it a try? I promise you that I will not let you fall!' He hemmed and hawed, but finally emphatically said, 'Yes! Let's do it!'"

"'Let's practice getting out of your chair, OK?' I asked him. We practiced three times. I asked if he was ready to take a few steps. He again said yes. He was gaining confidence. This time, the therapist gave him a cane. We walked a few steps. He had a giant smile on his face. I asked if he was ready to walk into the meeting. He almost hollered, YES!"

"We slowly walked to the closed door where the meeting was taking place. Unbeknownst to me, Delray's wife was taking minutes at the meeting. I knocked on the door and cracked it open. Delray and the therapist were behind me. I said, 'I have an announcement to make.' Everyone looked up. I said, 'I want you to meet the new Delray. Ta da!' I moved out of the way and Delray walked in. His wife actually screamed out, 'Delray, you're walking!' Everyone applauded and yelled, 'Way to go Delray!' His wife was crying. Delray was crying. Tears and smiles were running rampant. What a great moment. It's one that will be etched in my memory forever."

Bill's speaking engagements connected him with several stroke survivors' groups around the San Diego community, including Grossmont's Comebackers Club.

THE COMEBACKERS CLUB

"The Comebackers Club is a group of stroke survivors or people who have had a brain attack or traumatic brain injury," recreational therapist, Mary Williams, explained to us,

> We meet every month. We have a president, then a vice president, and the treasurer. We have people who help with fundraising. We have a board of survivors then meets every month, and we plan the activities, and we divide up the work. My role is as sensitively as possible to let them run as much as they can, but then also, because they have brain injuries, they do need assistance. There's an occupational therapist, Tina, and myself. We're the advisers of the club, and we help guide these individuals to help run the club.

> The club once a year does a meeting with its members. They announce it, and they talk about, "What's it going to be? What's your needs? What are the needs of the group?" They try to do a needs assessment, and we have a meeting, people bring up ideas of what they would really like to hear about. Once we get that, then the role of the board is to help facilitate in the next year our meetings based off of what they said.

> They also do have some big events, like we have a Christmas party every year. We have a Comebacker every year awards function where we recognize somebody that has exhibited the qualities of feeling engaged in their recovery, and having a sense of humor, meeting some of their goals that they had in their recovery, and that they helped make a difference in other people's lives. We do a Thanksgiving luncheon for those individuals and it's a great celebration for people who really don't have the family or the means to do anything.

As far as Mary could remember, she first met Bill when he agreed to come speak at a Comebacker's meeting. Fellow stroke survivor James Geter was in the audience that day. He tells us the story of how Bill inspired him to not only move into recovery but to become passionate about being a stroke advocate.

***

"Yes, that was my first visit to the club," James interjects, taking over the interview from Mary Williams. He's been listening attentively as we questioned the recreational therapist, but now seems anxious to jump in and share his own story. "I had a stroke in a summer of 2008," James continues. "I got released from the rehab just before my birthday, August 31, 2008. I never could get my balance to walk. I already had been a double amputee.[3] I couldn't get my balance to walk. Man, my life is over. In January, they decided to do an operation on my cerebellum."

"To help with your balance," Sarah nods, verbalizing her understanding.

"Then I had my balance back, and the therapist told my caregiver, 'Don't let him come in the wheelchair no more. He can walk.' I'm all, 'Man, you won't take me up to therapy in a wheelchair? I got to walk?'" The James's face crinkles as he pouts, pantomiming the frustration he'd felt at being denied an easy way out. He adopts a higher, feminine voice as he recounts his therapist's nagging: 'You said you was going to go to one of these Comebacker meetings. Way back in August, you said you was going to go to one of these meetings. I told you, you ought to go. You said you was going to go.'"

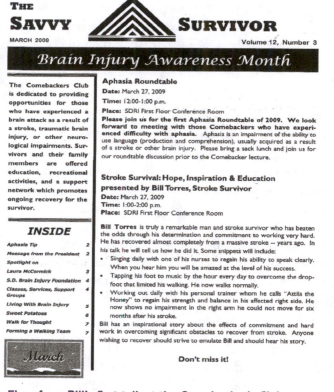

THE
SAVVY SURVIVOR
MARCH 2009   Volume 12, Number 3

Brain Injury Awareness Month

The Comebackers Club is dedicated to providing opportunities for those who have experienced a brain attack as a result of a stroke, traumatic brain injury, or other neurological impairments. Survivors and their family members are offered education, recreational activities, and a support network which promotes ongoing recovery for the survivor.

INSIDE

Aphasia Tip	2
Message from the President	2
Spotlight on Laura McCormick	3
S.D. Brain Injury Foundation	4
Classes, Services, Support Groups	4
Living With Brain Injury	5
Sweet Potatoes	6
Walk for Thought	7
Forming a Walking Team	7

March

Aphasia Roundtable
Date: March 27, 2009
Time: 12:00-1:00 p.m.
Place: SDRI First Floor Conference Room
Please join us for the first Aphasia Roundtable of 2009. We look forward to meeting with those Comebackers who have experienced difficulty with aphasia. Aphasia is an impairment of the ability to use language (production and comprehension), usually acquired as a result of a stroke or other brain injury. Please bring a sack lunch and join us for our roundtable discussion prior to the Comebacker lecture.

Stroke Survival: Hope, Inspiration & Education presented by Bill Torres, Stroke Survivor
Date: March 27, 2009
Time: 1:00-2:00 p.m.
Place: SDRI First Floor Conference Room

Bill Torres is truly a remarkable man and stroke survivor who has beaten the odds through his determination and commitment to working very hard. He has recovered almost completely from a massive stroke -- years ago. In his talk he will tell us how he did it. Some snippets will include:

- Singing daily with one of his nurses to regain his ability to speak clearly. When you hear him you will be amazed at the level of his success.
- Tapping his foot to music by the hour every day to overcome the drop-foot that limited his walking. He now walks normally.
- Working out daily with his personal trainer whom he calls "Attila the Honey" to regain his strength and balance in his affected right side. He now shows no impairment in the right arm he could not move for six months after his stroke.

Bill has an inspirational story about the effects of commitment and hard work in overcoming significant obstacles to recover from stroke. Anyone wishing to recover should strive to emulate Bill and should hear his story.

Don't miss it!

Flyer from Bill's first talk at the Comebacker's Club

Contributed by Mary Williams. Copyright © Kendall Hunt Publishing Company.

---

3. James's first leg was amputated in December of 2006 and his second leg was amputated in June 2007, both as a consequence of his diabetes. This made his recovery from his June 2008 stroke even more complex; he had to relearn to walk using two prosthetic legs.

Interview contributed by James Geter. Copyright © Kendall Hunt Publishing Company.

"I went in there with my walker, and I see Bill. The meeting had already started. Everybody in there was just like me—not perfect people. So, I just felt comfortable and walked in there with my walker. I'm sitting down with my caregiver listening to Bill. After a while, I ask 'Did he say he had a stroke?' 'Shut up, James, listen.'" We laugh as James re-enacts the sense of incredulity he felt as he watched this seemingly able-bodied man describe how he finally moved one finger after an eternity of trying. "After the meeting, I went up to Bill and I just asked 'Did you have a stroke?' 'Oh, yes, James, I had a stroke.' See, I wouldn't have never known he had a stroke. That's how I want to be. Just like that Bill."

James tells us how he began to attend more Comebacker meetings, and eventually took on more formal roles in the club. "Well, basically, I work at this barbecue, and I make calls," he begins.

"James comes in and he volunteers for the rehab barbecue," Mary elaborates. "We have a patient rehab barbecue every week and James and Dusty are our peer visitors. They come in and just help with the barbecue and visit with the patients' families and are sources of constant encouragement. Sometimes, James talks about how, at home, he might be feeling down and having one of his worst days. When he comes in here, we don't know that. He's got his happy face on and he is encouraging everybody and being that role model just like Bill does."

James flashes us a sparkling white grin from under the shadows of his baseball cap; it's easy to imagine how his optimism would be infectious. He talks to us about how he has begun to view everyday encounters as opportunities for advocacy, meeting stroke survivors and their family members on the streets, recruiting them to Comebackers, and even offering advice for making it to the meetings using San Diego's public transportation system. "I was in the rehab the last three weeks, and I couldn't wait to get out of there. Other patients asked, 'Why? You're getting treated hand-to-foot in here.' I told them, 'I get it, but I do have a life.' Man, I came to a couple meetings on a day pass."

"He was recently hospitalized in post-acute rehab for the last weeks," Mary translates for us, "he's talking about the fact that he would check himself out and come to our meetings."

"I got to go for our meeting. I got to go make my calls. People's counting on me," James emphasizes. Clearly, the Comebackers Club has given him a deep sense of purpose—the feeling that he is needed motivates him to push through his own health challenges.

"We have a big event coming up in August, and my goal is to really invite everybody I can to that," James continues. "Because, to me, that will sell you. When you get there, you see 80 people just like you. Whereas at home, you're watching TV, and all the actors are in excellent shape. With strangers, they have no idea, so they can treat you in a way that you don't deserve. Our group, we have an idea. Yes. They tell you, 'Keep your chin up, you got this, don't worry about this.' You hear that in our group. In the streets, you won't hear that."

"One of the questions that you asked earlier," Mary breaks in, "You asked, 'What are the challenges of being an effective peer mentor?'"

"Yes, I'd like to hear your perspective on that," Sarah says.

"From my perspective, I have so many stroke survivors that come to us and say, 'I want to be a peer visitor.' In selecting peer visitors for our program, we don't entertain really anybody that's within 18 months of their stroke because that period is a huge learning curve. They're going through so many emotions themselves. We encourage them to get involved in the club, come to this, start getting back involved in things."

"Then, not everybody has the personality for being a peer visitor. A peer visitor needs to be somebody who has empathy—it isn't all about themselves. James could come in and tell you two hours of stories about his personal life, but he doesn't do that. It's not about him."

"A peer visitor, their number one thing is to listen, is to observe where they are. It's not about James's ego. It's not about saying, '*I've* recovered *this* well.' It's about the person that's sitting across from them—the survivor or the caregiver."

"James is out there encouraging people, but you can't force it on people. But, you can give that listening ear. You can meet them where they're at. You can help guide them into their journey of recovery and get them signed up for information that will come to their house—information that maybe they'll never read until the sixth month of recovery, when they are ready for it."

"My peer visitors come from all areas," Mary continues. "We have people who are retired pilots from the military to captains in the navy to somebody who maybe didn't go to college. Everybody's life is very different. But the common theme is that they care about somebody else. At the moment when they're doing peer visits, they care more about somebody else than they do themselves. That's why James is such an inspiration to people—just like Bill was to him."

***

"I'm always thinking of titles for the book," Bill tells us, glancing over at Patricia in the passenger seat as he ferries us home from our meeting with Mary and James in his red Fiat. "One of the titles I was thinking of is *Echoes of a Stroke Survivor*. Because they reverberate—all of these stories reverberate. Everyone that I talk to, I say, 'Now, you're thanking me, but here is a way you can really thank me. You've got to talk to three people that have had strokes.'"

"Pay it forward," Sarah supplies from the back seat.

Bill nods. "I don't know if they do, but James has."

FALLING IN LOVE WITH THE PROCESS: CULTIVATING RESILIENCE IN HEALTH CRISES

CLOSING REFLECTIONS

In these stories of advocacy and interviews with those who have witnessed Bill's advocacy work, we learn several key lessons about what makes his approach to working with stroke survivors effective. These include factors like Bill's ability to remember and draw on his own experiences to empathize with stroke survivors, the value of identifying the source of a person's motivation (i.e., being able to hold a baby) and tailoring a messaging accordingly, and the importance of putting aside their own story to actively listen to another person's fears, hopes, and needs. Additionally, interviews with a recreational therapist and other health care administrators highlight the limitations of existing stroke rehabilitation services in the United States and underline the vital importance of community resources and peer mentors like Bill. In Chapter 13, we describe the ways in which Bill engages in advocacy work that extends his impact beyond the more formal channels of hospital programs.

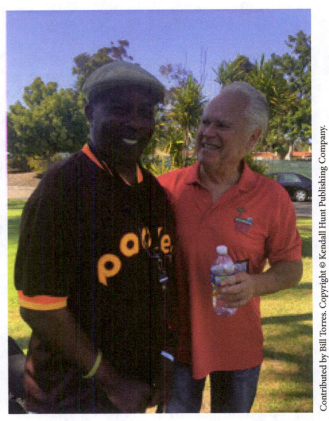

James and Bill

CHAPTER 13

Becoming an "Independent Contractor": Advocating Beyond the Hospital

"Bill is an independent contractor," Alvarado Hospital's recreational therapist, Mary Williams, explains. "The unique thing about Bill is that Bill will go out and can travel and go anywhere. We're tied liability-wise with our peer visitors; we can do our visits here at the hospital or at a sanctioned hospital event. But, to actually go out and do a visit … we don't go to the homes just because of our hospital's liability. Bill is just so flexible—he goes anywhere people need him."

Mary's comments highlight one of the valuable aspects of an "independent contractor" like Bill. Unconstrained by the bureaucracy of the healthcare system, Bill is free to pursue relationships with fellow stroke survivors in more intimate ways—in their homes, using his personal phone number—often making the most of chance encounters with individuals (and their family members) seeking guidance along the long road of recovery. In this chapter, we explore the ways that Bill pursued opportunities for advocacy beyond official, hospital-sanctioned program, including interactions with people who e-mail him through his personal website, people who call him directly from other states or countries, and interactions with students through his presentations in college classrooms.

ADVOCACY VIA THE WORLD WIDE WEB

As stroke advocacy became a central feature of Bill's life, he began to seek alternative ways to connect with others who might benefit from his story. He developed his own website, writing a summary of his own experiences and curating a hodge-podge collection of photos—pictures of health care providers who were an important part of his journey, snapshots of dear friends, black-and-white photos of his childhood and young adulthood, and photographs of his beloved ducks. The result is a website that offers an endearingly intimate digital scrapbook that feels as warmly open and straightforward as its creator. Bill included his personal e-mail and phone number on the site as well as a guestbook, hoping to hear from other stroke survivors and their family members. And he did. Bill estimates that his website received over 6,000 hits from people located around the country. Some contacts even came from the other side of the globe, including one memorable phone call from London.

STROKE ADVOCACY STORY: SORUNKEB (TUNDE) OF NIGERIA

"One afternoon while trying to solve the *New York Times* crossword puzzle, my phone rang. Or I should say, it quacked," Bill jests.

"I answered the phone with a 'good afternoon.' A voice with a thick accent and a distinct mumble attempted to say hello. The call was from London, England. The person said his name was Tunde and he wanted to speak to Bill Torres. This took a few times because of his accent and the effects of a stroke. We spoke for over an hour. What I deciphered was that he was from Nigeria, but he was working on a project in London. His mother was very worried about him. He needed to get better so that he could return to Nigeria."

"Tunde and I had a series of conversations. We discussed his therapy and I gave him a few exercises to help him in his quest to get better. I used music and singing—singing to help his speech and music to help his leg and arm. 'Just sit, closing your eyes and tapping your foot in your mind. It helps to make the new connections in the brain,' I told him. 'Same thing with your hands and fingers.'"

"After about two months he was ready to go home. I wished him well and told him to please keep me informed on his progress. He was a very determined man. With his drive and determination, I knew he would heal quickly."

"'Quack, quack,' went the phone, and I answered. It was Tunde. He said someone wanted to talk to me. I heard, 'Hello this is Tunde's Mother.' She broke out in sobs and thanked me profusely. I said she had a wonderful and courageous son. Tunde said thanks to me—they were walking together along the beach. The three of us cried together and said our goodbyes."

"A few months later I received an e-mail from Tunde. Turns out he is a chief of a village and was working in London on some water machines. It's the first time his village has running water. I thought, *What a wonderful story and I'm glad I played a little part of it.*"

***

Clearly, Bill's homespun website allowed him to make some meaningful connections with stroke survivors in some surprisingly far-flung places. He met Sally, a young woman who lived near a lake in Maine and had connected with images of Bill at his duck pond. She contacted him to ask for his advice to support her mother. Once, she called Bill just so that he could hear the mournful cry of the loons on one muggy summer evening. Bill met Emilio, a Sergeant from Chile who feared that he would be discharged from the Marines because he could not no longer salute. The masculine military man was uncharacteristically emotional when he called Bill after several weeks, reporting that he was nearly ready to go back on duty.

Yet some of Bill's most impactful advocacy work was not with distant stroke survivors. In fact, it was not with stroke survivors at all. Rather, it was the work that brought him back to in touch with a group he had worked with once before, several careers ago—students. After meeting Patricia and Assistant Professor of Rehabilitation Counseling, Mark Tucker, Bill recognized that his story of recovery might be used to inspire future generations of health professionals, caregivers, and—potentially—advocates.

ADVOCACY VIA THE COLLEGE CLASSROOM

Patricia arrives at Dr. Tucker's office to find his door ajar. She taps lightly and a man, dressed smartly in light blue slacks and dress shirt, appears at the door. "You must be Patricia," he says. "Come on in and have a seat."

"Thank you, Mark. We really appreciate your time in offering your perspective of Bill Torres," Patricia offers as she looks around at the sun-filled, neatly organized office.

"I am so happy to help. Bill has offered so much to me and my students. They just love him. He really makes a difference," Mark gushes a bit, clearly enamored with Bill.

"Fantastic. I know you don't have a lot of time, so let's get started. First, I'd just like you tell me who you are and what you do here at San Diego State," Patricia says. She carefully positions her iPhone on Dr. Tucker's desk so that the its microphone will be more likely to pick up his soften-spoken commentary. Patricia is interviewing solo today as Sarah prepares to teach her own college classes on the opposite side of the country in Winter Park, Florida.

"I'm Mark Tucker," Mark begins, "I'm an Assistant Professor in the Administration, Rehabilitation, and Postsecondary Education department. Within that department we have a couple of different emphases. One is in postsecondary education leadership and one is in rehabilitation counseling. I teach across both, but my background is more in rehabilitation counseling. What we're really focused on there is training counselors to work with people with disabilities, primarily around securing and retaining employment. That might mean going to work for the first time after growing up with a disability, or it might mean getting back to work after incurring a disability or multiple disabilities."

"Great," Patricia says. "Let me ask you this question first of all: Can you tell me the story of when you first met Bill?"

"OK, sure. I teach a class—it's actually a two-semester class—on medical and psychological aspects of disabilities for counselors studying in our graduate program in rehabilitation counseling. That class is actually held at Sharp Rehabilitation, a working rehab facility. I make use of a lot of guest presenters who come in and know more about a particular topic than I do. We draw heavily on folks at Sharp. Therapists, physicians, community health educators—that type of thing."

"So, I was talking with a woman there who is the Administrative Assistant to the Director. She was saying to me, 'You really have to meet Bill because he would be great in your class.' I usually try to bring in folks who have a medical background, but who also maybe have lived experience with a disability or are involved in some other way. That way, the class is not all just medicine, medicine, medicine."

"I called him up—I think I e-mailed him actually," Mark continues, breaking into a smile. "I don't know if you've noticed this, but if I send him an e-mail I usually get a reply within an hour."

"It's true," Patricia laughs, "he's so quick."

"Yes, he is," Mark agrees. "I e-mailed him and I said, 'Here's the situation. The physician up at Sharp, the Medical Director, Dr. Stenehjem, is coming into my class. He talks about the clinical aspects of stroke and I would like somebody to come and talk about some of the other parts of stroke. What life's like after surviving a stroke?' He was like, 'Yeah, I'll be there.'"

"Dr. Stenehjem comes in and talks for about the first half of the class," Mark continues, narrating what has become the routine structure for this visit. "Then, Bill comes in and watches the tail end of Dr Stenehjem's talk, then talks about his perspective as a survivor. I was thinking back about this, and I think it was about eight years ago, the first time he came to the class."

"Wow. So, does he come in every year, then?" Patricia follows up.

"Every year," Mark nods. "Usually it's in the fall, so I contact him during the summer and I say, 'Bill are you up for coming in the fall?' He's like, 'I'll be there.' I always worry when I bring folks in year after year, am I going to wear them out? Am I imposing on their time too much?"

Patricia laughs, trying—and failing—to imagine Bill ever running out of energy or time for an experience like this. "He's such a good storyteller," she comments.

"He is," Mark laughs. "That class runs from 4:00 to 6:40 p.m. and then some of the students have seven o'clock classes, so we wrap a little early. He wants to keep going—he's just so passionate about it. It's not like you have to put the brakes on him in a hard manner, but it's like, 'OK, some of these students have to go!'"

"He pays a lot of attention to the room and to the people in the room," Mark adds. "He'll refer to people—students in the class. He'll just start having a conversation with them. He's got what I would call, like a forceful personality, but not a domineering personality. If he's in the room, you know it and he's going to command some attention, but by including people, not by elevating himself."

"Yesss," Patricia says, drawing out the "s" in her enthusiastic endorsement of this character assessment. "That really makes sense. How would you describe his impact on your students?" Patricia follows up, thinking of Bill's visits to her own classroom.

"I think initially students are just kind of impressed with him personally, right?" Mark replies, cradling his chin with one hand and squinting as he thinks. "But also, when he was sort of at the tail end his recovery, he was kind of presented with a decision: 'Do I go to work, or do I commit my life to helping others?' He put aside the closet full of nice suits. He elected to dedicate his time and his efforts to helping other people."

"These are students who are doing that as well," Mark continues, connecting Bill's work to his students' passions. "They're either already in the field or they're getting ready to enter the field. It's a helping profession. They're going to be paid for what they're doing, but they're going to work at a discounted price, relative to what they could get if they worked in banking or something like that, right? So, they're foregoing some of the material rewards for maybe good karma," Mark chuckles, amused by his own, idealistic description of rehabilitation counseling as a career path. "Bill kind of exemplifies that in a more striking manner," he continues, "He's foregoing any kind of an income at all, basically, and committing himself to doing this kind of work. I think that really resonates with folks and that has an impact on them."

"The other thing is, that a lot of students will disclose that they have a family member who's had a stroke," Mark adds. "Bill has given out his e-mail, his website has his personal phone number and stuff like that. Who puts his personal number on the website?" Mark laughs. "That's part of his old-school nature again. He'll tell me, 'Call me at two in the morning, call me at three in the morning.' I don't want my students calling me at three in the morning," Mark jokes, one eyebrow raised skeptically. "I appreciate them, I love talking to them, but I'm not going to give them my cell phone." Patricia nods sympathetically, imagining hundreds of her undergraduate students sending panicked end-of-semester texts asking for extra credit. "A smaller number of students, they'll actually contact him," Mark reports. "They'll see if they can get him to talk to a family member who may be struggling."

"Has Bill had any impact on you, personally?" Patricia follows up, pushing further.

"Of course," Mark laughs. "On a very practical level, it's wonderful to have him as a resource. He's always trying to get a little bit more information to the students. He'll say, 'I've got this other DVD called *Still Me* that I think is really good. I'll get you a copy, Mark. Load it up for the students if they want it. His level of investment in students who he's only going to meet one time?" Mark shakes his head, impressed. "He's got a lot of faith that he's going to have an impact on them through that really brief interaction—and he does. That's another way he has a bit of an impact on me—just seeing his optimism around and what he can do to have a positive impact on people in a really short period of time."

"It's one of the things that I think is really nice about the profession I'm working in." Mark's normally soften-spoken tone softens further as he reflects on the nature of his own life's work. "The people that you come into contact with … I feel like that's part of that karma. You get to meet some really nice folks, and some folks who are just remarkable. Maybe this is just bias, but I feel like in my field, the proportion you meet of those remarkable people is a bit higher. Getting to meet Bill and interact with him is some of that payback for trying to do good stuff. It makes working in this field really enjoyable. It's good to see him every year, and just to know that he's out there—having a positive impact."

***

"I spoke to Addie's class the other day," Bill reports, referencing the recent guest lecture he did for Patricia's colleague at San Diego State, Professor Addie Winslow. Bill's voice, a bit tinny and distorted on Patricia's speaker phone, sounds uncharacteristically tentative. "I'm not sure I really did my best," he continues. "I've been feeling a little weird—mentally—lately. I'm finding that my emotions are just all out of whack, and the words just aren't coming out smoothly. They're lingering symptoms from my stroke—just like that weird, random burning I've been having in my tongue lately. Anyway," Bill sighs, "I don't think it went very well in Addie's class."

"I'm sure that you were great," Patricia reassures. Her brow furrows; this anxious, self-doubting version of Bill is so different from the relentlessly positive, charismatic Bill she has become accustomed to. Yet this experience of suddenly feeling insecure in the classroom is familiar; academics often go through stages of imposter syndrome,[1] questioning their own ability and authority to speak even about their own specialized knowledge. "I tell you what," Patricia says, "Let me see if Addie is willing to collect some feedback from her students. I'm sure your talk went better than you think it did."

When the students' comments roll in, they reflect the powerful ways in which Bill's presence inspires students not only to learn about—and act to prevent—stroke but also to emulate his commitment to supporting others:

---

1. Imposter syndrome—sensations of not belonging; feeling that one's competence and success are fundamentally fraudulent and inauthentic (Breeze, 2018).

Bill spoke today about his experience with a life-altering stroke (actually 12 of them) that he uses as a catalyst for the healing of other people. He said a quote that I wrote down and will stick with me for a while, if not forever: 'I learned to fall in love with the process of healing.'

I enjoyed this quote as well as his infectious energy because going through recovery for an eating disorder entails the same mindset. For me, Bill's story hit home because I myself am going through intense healing that take daily practice and mental commitment. He inspired me to really embrace whatever stage of life we are in because it only lasts for so long.

Aside from recovering himself, he is able to channel all that he has learned into helping fellow stroke survivors get a second chance at life. I hope to do the same thing Bill does because I know it only takes one person to make an immense difference in someone's life.

—Brielle

Bill's story, in general, was very motivating. He reminded me, directly and passionately, that 'not giving-up' is a key to change lives. Some classmates asked questions regarding exercise and strokes. I am more interested in his willpower. If he came back, I'd ask: did he ever think about giving up the exercise during his recovery?

—Zhongfeng

To me, Bill's sheer desire to live the life he wanted was what I enjoyed most from his talk: for the first time in a while, I got to witness a very successful person who got there from sheer willpower, cooperation, and kindness to others. The fact that Bill not only recovered, but went back into the hospitals to sincerely help others day in and day out—whereas many others would want to 'get on' with their lives—transcends what I thought real people could truly do. He just has so much heart and I admire that enormously; It has driven me to try and have some heart of my own.

—Analise

When I was younger, I volunteered at a healthcare facility for elderly patients. I think it was hard for me to relate to their struggles and I had to change my communication style to tend to their needs. I also did not have a connection that demonstrated that I know where they were coming from. I think it is really special for patients to have someone like Bill to encourage them and show patients that they can make it out of their situation as well.

—Adam

My family member had a 'mini-stroke' a couple years ago. Getting that phone call was the scariest thing I've experienced yet, waiting for results was even harder because your mind just goes to that dark place. Hearing your story, especially your resilience and gratitude for life, really hits home and reminds me how important attitude, support, and preparations are. Keep inspiring, pushing, advocating and fighting for those who can't.

—Amal

Our world needs more people like Bill. Bill is like a fire in a fire place, he helped to light up many candles with hope. If Bill comes back, I would like to say, 'you're the fire for many people. Thank you.'

—Valente

My family member experienced a stroke several years ago and has yet to recover. He lays in a hospital bed in the living room and has affected my family in so many ways. My question to you is, how can someone help support them through what they are going through?

—Brianne

I try to make a difference, too, but sometimes I feel drained and discouraged. But, overall, I have hope—and you made me feel very hopeful. One day I promise to come down to the duck pond and look for the guy with the biggest smile. I'll say hello.

—Jordan

> *When I die one day, I hope I return as duck. I'll land in the lake that you visit every day. Free breakfast would be a great deal for a duck!*
>
> —Beth

Before every semester that she teaches Communication 321: Health Communication, Patricia works diligently for months contacting potential speakers for her class. Her goal is to have a wide range of speakers on a diverse set of topics. In addition to Bill's presentation, students have enjoyed presentations by family physicians, midwives, end-of-life therapists, gerontologists, oncologists, hospice staff, acupuncturists, and nonprofits devoted to ending youth violence, assisting women who struggle with eating disorders, addictions, or intimate partner violence, and others. Yet, every semester, when Patricia asks students who their favorite speaker was that semester, it is always Bill Torres. There is just something that clicks for students and that touches them deeply when they see and hear Bill, an SDSU graduate from over 50 years ago. Bill is not intimidated by a class of 200 students in a big lecture hall. Instead, he sees it as an opportunity to convince as many young people as he can that they need to know about stroke and what it takes to survive—even thrive after stroke.

CLOSING REFLECTIONS

From the time he felt capable of reaching out to others after his stroke until today, more than a decade later, Bill seeks out any opportunity to reach out to others through his story. As an "independent contractor" Bill is not constrained by the rules and regulations embedded in hospital systems. He is free to reach out—through his website, presentations in college classrooms, and spontaneous conversations with others (on the street, in grocery store lines, and in restaurants). Opportunities come to Bill in e-mails or phone calls from people across the United States, and even from other countries. He frequently receives calls from people who learned about him from students he's talked to or from other stroke survivors he has worked with.

Yet, while these last two chapters have shared positive stories of the rewarding encounters Bill has participated in, he still struggles emotionally when people don't follow through on his advice for recovery or don't keep in touch to update him on their progress. In Chapter 14, we explore the complexities of engaging in this kind of work—including the emotional challenges it entails.

REFERENCE

Breeze M. (2018). Imposter syndrome as a public feeling. In Y. Taylor & K. Lahad (Eds.), *Feeling academic in the neoliberal university: Feminist flights, fights and failures* (pp. 191–219). Cham, Switzerland: Palgrave-Macmillan.

CHAPTER 14

Bill steers his nimble red Fiat down a Mission Valley exit ramp, guiding it around the curve. We're shadowing him today as he completes a house call; he's excited for us to meet one of the stroke survivors he's been working with recently. "Back to the stroke protocol," Bill says, returning to a topic he has discussed with us repeatedly. "Everything is done physically. The stroke is *the brain*. Why don't we have someone working on the brain?"

"It costs money," he continues, answering his own question. "Everything is physical to get you in and out of the hospital so that they can move on to the next patient. That's very frustrating for me. Your *brain* is broken! But they don't give you any psychological elements in your treatment. Going back to John and Marsha …." Bill pauses, glancing over at Patricia in the passenger seat, "Did I tell you that story?"

"You gave us a typed story with that title, but we haven't heard you tell it yet," Sarah offers from the back seat.

"It started out like any other day," Bill begins, shifting quickly into story mode. "I drove out to the lake to feed the birds and squirrels. When I pulled into my parking place, there was Phillip the Goose waiting for me. I got out of the car and opened the hatchback to get out the food. Phillip was honking, and the squirrels were hovering around my feet, begging for peanuts." Sarah laughs, imagining Phillip wagging his tail feathers in anxious anticipation of his daily birdseed feast.

"Then, it happened," Bill continues with his usual dramatic flair. "My phone starts quacking. I wonder who is calling me so early at 6:45 a.m. I didn't recognize the number, but I tell people that they can call me anytime. So, I answer with a 'good morning.' Wow, what a response! The female, in a desperate, screaming voice says, 'Help, he's trying to kill me!'"

Patricia gasps, listening raptly as Bill turns down a wide, palm tree-lined street.

"I said, 'Hang up and call 911!' She was breathing heavily and kept repeating he's trying to kill me. I asked her to calm down, take a big breath and release it—breathe, breathe. After a few minutes of breathing in and out she seemed to calm down. She said, 'No. You've got to help me. They told me at the American Heart Association that you could help me.'

'Oh, your husband had a stroke?' I guessed.

'Yes.'

'And he's trying to kill you?'

'Yes.'

'Where is he?'

'He's in the front room.'

I said, 'Oh, I don't think he's trying to kill you. Why don't you calm down? Count to ten and then re-start.'

She says, 'We get into these arguments. It's so frustrating. *He's* so frustrating.'

I asked her if I could possibly talk to her husband. She calls out, 'John, Mr. Torres wants to talk to you!'

A few seconds pass. Then I hear a 'hello,' with a slight trace of a slur—a sign of speech aphasia.

'Hi, my name is Bill. To whom am I speaking?'

'This is John.'

'John, tell me what's happening.'

'She's crazy, I'm not trying to kill her.'

'Then why is she making that accusation?'

'She's mad because we had an argument at breakfast.'

'John, let me speak to your wife.'

John put his wife, Marsha, back on the phone and I said, 'Why don't I come up and see him? Is that okay? Ask him if it's okay.'

She goes, 'John, can Bill come out and see you? He is a stroke survivor.'

He says, 'Sure. Why not?'

'OK give me your address and I'll be up as soon as the traffic lets up. Let's say about 10:30. Is that OK?' She gives me the address and we hang up.

While driving to their house I started thinking about the possibilities of what may be happening. I know from experience that I would sometimes have word displacement, meaning that I would call something a different name. For example, I would call 'Michael' 'George.' I knew his name was Michael, but when I tried to say 'Michael' it would always come out 'George.' For many words, I had to use substitute words because I knew the word just wouldn't come out right. Marsha said that their arguments were usually at meal times. A light went off in my head—I thought I knew the problem. I had encountered this before, but not with the dramatics.

I pulled up to the house and got out of my car. Marsha was standing on the porch waiting for me. 'I'm Bill,' I introduced myself. 'What seems to be the problem?'

She says, 'Every morning it's always an argument.'

I said, 'Let me go talk to him.'

I went in. He's reading the paper. I said, 'Hey John, I'm Bill. You had a stroke?'

'Yes.'

I was aware that John's right side was affected. I asked John if he had an ischemic stroke on the left part of the brain. He said yes. He was about 50 pounds overweight and lacked mobility. We discussed his stroke and all the ramifications that came with it. After his hospitalization and his physical and occupational therapy sessions were over, he quit therapy altogether. This happens too many times—some stroke survivors just give up!

I said, 'You're arguing a lot with your wife, John?'

He says, 'Yes. The old bitch, she gets me so mad.'

'When does this usually happen?' I had an inkling of what was happening.

'It's always at breakfast time,' Marsha says.

I knew what it was right then. He had a—I don't know the term for it. I think it's 'transference.' Word transference. When he asked for the salt, he would say ketchup. So, she'd pass him the ketchup and he'd say, 'No, no, no! I want the ketchup.' She'd go, 'This *is* the ketchup.' 'No, that's not the ketchup,' he'd say, and then he'd grab the salt: '*This* is the ketchup!' And they'd argue back-and-forth about it."

"Mmm," Sarah backchannels from the back seat, picturing Bill's impromptu role as marriage counselor extraordinaire in the midst of a husband-wife spat.

"I said, 'Just a minute, John. Let me go talk to your wife,'" Bill continues, adopting the even-paced, eminently reasonable-sounding tone he must have used that day. "I went out to the porch and said, 'Marsha, I know what's wrong. When he wants you to pass something, you give him that thing and it's the wrong thing all the time.'

'He asked for the ketchup and I give him the ketchup!' Marsha says, throwing her hands in the air.

I said, 'I understand. So, let me explain to you what happens.' I told her about word transference. I got thinking, *How can I defuse this?* I said, 'Marsha, I'm going to ask you a question right now. You don't have to answer me. But if you answer me, I need the truth,' I said, 'I'll go no further than here. Do you love your husband?'

You could see a jolt in her body. 'Yes. Yes, I love my husband.'

'OK. Stay here.' I went in and asked the same thing of John, and he said 'yes,' too. I said, 'OK. I think I can help this.'

I called Marsha in. I sat them down at the table. I put some items on the table: 'Give me the ketchup. Give me the salt. Put things on there.' I said, 'Now John, when you want something on this table, I want you to preface it with *Marsha, I love you. Would you please pass the ketchup?* And Marsha, you say to John, *I love you too, John. Is this what you want?* and you pick up the ketchup and you hand it to him. John, if that's not what you want, you just say, *Marsha, I love you, but I really want the ketchup.* Now, Marsha, you'd say, *OK, John. I love you too. Is this what you want?* and pick things until you find the right thing for him.' I said, 'Would you do that for me? Let's practice.' I practiced that. Then, I left them.

A couple of weeks later, Martha calls and she says, 'Oh, we haven't argued and I really feel good. Thank you, Bill.'

I said, 'Well, that's wonderful. Call me up every once in a while and check in. I want to know how you are.'

Two months pass, and she calls and says, 'We're arguing again.'

'Why are you arguing again?'

'We got tired of telling each other we love them.'"

We crack up together at the punchline of Bill's story, just as his cell phone erupts with the familiar quacking ringtone.

"That's Randy," Bill says, naming the videographer he met while doing advocacy work with Sharp.[1] We've just met Randy several days ago, interviewing him about his work with Bill.

"Go ahead and get it," Patricia encourages as Bill places the phone on speaker mode.

"Randy?" Bill picks up. "Good morning, sir! Hey, hey, I'm with Patricia and Sarah right now. They tell me all about you—I don't believe it, but they tell me." We can hear Randy's good-natured laughter on the other end of the phone line. "Say good morning," Bill instructs us.

"Hi, Randy," Sarah calls from the backseat.

"Hello! What's happening? You guys are becoming stalkers," Randy quips.

"I know," Sarah says as Patricia jokes, "That's our job! We're professionals."

"We always wanted two girls as stalkers, though," Randy parries.

"How are you, Randy?" Bill asks, "I haven't talked to you for a few days."

"I know, I've just been on my next big project. Would you have time to go to Shakespeare's at 11?" Randy asks, naming a popular San Diego pub.

"No," Bill says, a hint of pride creeping into his voice, "Patricia and Sarah are going up with me to see Kate. They're going to watch me work."

∗∗∗

Bill's story about John and Marsha reads like a scene from a sitcom; a charmingly funny vignette of marital strife caused by fundamental challenges in communicating each other's needs. However, it serves as a useful case study for exploring the issues that Bill faces in navigating the tension-filled situations that his advocacy work often places him in. In this story, we observe how Bill draws on his personal experiences to understand the root of this couple's problem. He leverages his skills as a former teacher and salesman to validate and diffuse Marsha's frustrations, come up with a potential solution to the problem, secure consent and a sense of commitment from both husband and wife, and model more effective communication through role play. However, unlike some of Bill's other stories of advocacy, the John and Marsha story is not a straight-forward success. As he tells this tale,

---

1. Randy filmed Bill's life story for Sharp's Victories of Spirit Award; more about this in Chapter 15.

Bill begins to articulate the frustration he feels when he encounters stroke survivors who appear to have "given up" on their own rehabilitation. In addition, the John and Marsha story reveals that stroke survivors are embedded in a system of family and friends that do not always understand the ways their actions can be supportive and unsupportive. Efforts to work with a stroke survivor might not be successful when key support providers, such as family and friends, do not get on board with—or even undermine—strategies to address the survivor's recovery needs. In many cases, this occurs because they don't understand what stroke is or what the recovery process entails. Health care providers may not have worked directly with them to offer the knowledge they require to become the support that the survivor needs. In addition, it is not uncommon for caregivers to experience burnout, particularly when they do not take breaks from enacting the caregiver role.[2]

In this chapter, we discuss the challenges Bill faces in working with stroke survivors and their friends/family members who do not follow through on or implement his advice. Additionally, we consider instances where the communication strategies Bill employs might not always be well-suited to all survivors' communication preferences. Finally, we explore how unsuccessful or unsatisfying encounters affect Bill's mental health. Bill's encounters with Kate exemplify the emotional rollercoaster he experiences in working with fellow stroke survivors.

KATE

"How did you find out about Kate?" Patricia asks as Bill wraps up his phone call with Randy.

"My friend, Charlie, was in line at a Rite Aid pharmacy to get a prescription," Bill explains, "He struck up a conversation with this young lady and she said her mother had a stroke. 'Go call Bill,' he told her. So, she called me. I went up to see Kate at the group home where she lives, and that's how it started."

Patricia probes further as Bill pulls up to a stop light. "How long ago did she have that stroke?"

"It's almost two years. When I went over to see Kate, I said, 'Let me look at your hand. Would you mind if I take a picture of it? Has it been closed all this time?'"

"For two years?" Patricia clarifies, sounding shocked.

"Yes," Bill confirms. "It had never opened. She has an occupational therapist, but that's why I say that the protocol is all wrong. I was over, showed an occupational therapist these pictures of Kate's opened hand, and he went, 'Oh my God, this is great.' I didn't say it, but I thought, *Well, you guys could do this, it's simple.*"

---

2. *15 Things Caregivers Should Know After a Loved One Has Had a Stroke.* https://www.strokeassociation.org/en/help-and-support/for-family-caregivers/15-things-caregivers-should-know-after-a-loved-one-has-had-a-stroke

FALLING IN LOVE WITH THE PROCESS: CULTIVATING RESILIENCE IN HEALTH CRISES

"How old is Kate?" Patricia asks.

"62."

"She's young!"

"Yes. She has complete aphasia. I go over the vowels with her. She has a speech therapist, but I will work on it, too. I work on helping her to say, 'no.' I tell her, 'I know you're going to do this because all the women say no to me,'" Bill says, winking at Patricia before he continues. "Some people respond better than other people. Some people are afraid, and you can see sadness in their eyes. When you are a stroke survivor and people come and look at you, you immediately get into a defensive mood, even if you know they're not going to hurt you or do anything. Just the idea of people looking at me, I hated it. I felt like I was a leper."

"I wish I had taken pictures of Kate's eyes," Bill adds, his tone lightening. "Because eyes are the windows to the soul, and her eyes are getting brighter now than they were when I first met her. I've been with her eight times now. That's the most anyone's worked just with her hand."

"Bill, why do you think the hand so important?" Patricia asks.

"To me?" Bill navigates a left turn, silent for a moment as he formulates a response. "Because the hand starts everything, going all up the arm up to the shoulder. Once you start working the hand, once you start at the fingers, the brain starts getting the connections back. The connections have to go through the arm. The connections are affecting this arm, this elbow, this shoulder. Once you have that movement of opening your hand—it's wonderful."

"Yes," Patricia nods. "But it's not just a physical thing. I mean it *is* a physical thing, I'm hearing that," she clarifies. "But I'm also hearing that there's something psychologically important for us, as human beings, to be able to use our hands."

"Yes," Bill agrees as he guides the Fiat toward the curb, parking neatly. "That sets us apart from other animals. Our hands will grasp to pick things up or set things down. They'll reach out to shake another person's hand."

***

"Hi, Kate!" Bill's voice is characteristically warm and contagiously optimistic as he greets the regal-looking woman sitting in a black Lazy Boy in front of a flat screen television. When she looks up at us, her face seems surprisingly alert and relatively unlined—a sharp contrast to the elderly, stooped woman we had been imagining. She wears a hint of makeup, earrings, and a necklace. The teal color of her cardigan complements the white-blonde coloring of her straight, shoulder-length hair. "Let's sit down together at the dining room table," Bill suggests. He offers Kate his arm, lifting her from the cushions and guiding her toward a seat in the nearby, sunlight-filled room.

"Good to meet you, Kate," Patricia says as Sarah smiles a greeting. We had been worried that our visit might make Kate feel self-conscious and shy, but she appears open to our presence as we gather around the table; a slight smile curves one corner of her mouth.

Bill asks Kate for permission to work with her hand, waiting for the telltale nod of her head before gently grasping her fingers. He places her right hand on the table and begins a gradual process of kneading and unfurling. "See how her hand will curl back up when she pays attention to it?" Bill says. As soon as he calls Kate's attention to her fingers, they curl back in on themselves protectively. "It's much easier to work with them when she's distracted," he continues, resuming his massaging. "You should ask Kate where she's from," Bill suggests, a hint of mischief in his eyes, "You'll never guess."

"OK," Patricia says, rising to his challenge. "Are you from the West Coast, Kate?" She is careful to phrase her questions so that Kate can participate with yes/no responses, remembering what Bill had explained about how stroke survivors with aphasia might become frustrated with the challenge of articulating more complex responses. Kate shakes her head slightly; she's not a California native. "The East Coast?" Sarah tries. Head shake, *no.* "Midwest?" *no.* "South?" Kate nods slightly. We begin the process of trying to identify Kate's home state. "Georgia? Arkansas? Texas? Louisiana?" We keep naming states, racking our brains to conjure a map of the southern United States. Each guess receives another headshake from Kate—*no.*

Finally, Bill takes pity on us and offers a hint, lifting his left hand and pointing downward. "Further south? South America?" Sarah guesses. She is rewarded by Kate's slight head nod. We test our knowledge of geography further, naming countries in South America, Central America, and the Caribbean. "She's from Ecuador," Bill interjects, finally losing patience with our guessing game. "Before her stroke, Kate had a career as a Spanish-to-English translator. Actually, she translated between three different languages."

"Wow," Sarah says, impressed. She looks intently at the beautiful woman in front of her, imaging how difficult it would be to experience such severe aphasia after spending a lifetime fluently navigating multiple tongues.

"I used to know Spanish pretty well," Patricia says, seizing on this opportunity to connect with Kate. "I spent a sabbatical living in Costa Rica and interviewing healthcare providers about integrative medicine." Patricia pauses as she tries to recall some of the Spanish words and phrases that used to come so easily to her. "Yo … vive … en San Jose para seis meses," she attempts, struggling a bit with the verb conjugations. "Y mi esposo y mi hija, Makenna, fueron conmigo. Usted fue en San Jose?"[3] The ghost of a smile appears on Kate's lips as she nods her head, *yes.*

---

3. Patricia attempts to tell Kate that she lived in San Jose for 6 months and that her husband and her daughter, Makenna, went with her. She asks Kate if she had ever been to San Jose.

"Look at the difference in Kate's hand," Bill interrupts, calling our attention back to the work he has been doing during our chat.

"That's impressive," Patricia enthuses, noting that Kate's fingers—once curled tightly—now lay almost flat on the dining room table. Bill places Kate's right hand on a white piece of paper marked with today's date. He takes out a camera and snaps a picture to mark the progress they've made. "OK, Kate, we are done for today," Bill tells her. "I'll come back to visit you soon."

"Would you mind if I came back too, Kate?" Patricia inquires, looking directly into Kate's eyes. Another nod, *yes*.

***

"I'm so happy that you guys got to see and got to participate. I wish I could have you there all the time," Bill says as we climb back into the Fiat and buckle in. "Yes, that was wonderful, I'm telling you. You don't know how much …" Bill's voice is thick with sudden emotion. "It was 14 years ago that I had the stroke, and she's the first one that I have gotten to meet more than twice."

"Really?" Patricia raises her eyebrows, shocked.

"Yes. Everyone else since that day, they just walk away. They just don't want to do it; they don't have the time."

***

"The book is coming along!" Patricia says excitedly as we take our usual seats around her dining room table. Several weeks have passed since our visit with Kate, and we've been busily brainstorming, writing, and revising. We're excited to show Bill the progress we've made in outlining a potential structure for the chapters. "We actually have a copy of the outline of the book to share with you, Bill," Patricia adds, sliding a typed packet toward him across the polished oak tabletop. "There it is."

"Wonderful. All right," Bill says distractedly as he begins scanning our bullet-pointed ideas.

"We're still thinking about the title, and about what images we might include on the cover," Sarah adds. "We've been thinking about those pictures you took of Kate's hands, but we'd have to get her permission."

"Yes," Bill replies slowly, sounding suddenly forlorn. "I haven't heard from her. I called her up and left a message. She never called back. That makes me sad."

"Yes, it's hard," Patricia validates.

"It's almost like a death. I just feel just empty that it happened, you know? I'm forcible sometimes, but I try not to really force myself on people."

"As you know, they have to be ready," Patricia responds empathetically. "And some people just can't seem to get ready, can they?"

"I get really down. Sometimes I get depressed and I don't really want to see anybody because I feel like I'm wasting my time. I went to a psychologist, you know. Last week I was ready to call her up because I was dealing with someone that had a stroke. I had talked to this person before and they weren't getting any better. I asked them, 'are you doing this?' and they said, 'Oh, once in a while.' It's very difficult because they can always agree with you, but once you walk away they go back to the same thing."

'Well, it sounds to me Bill like …"

"That I'm crazy, huh?" Bill interrupts with a weak attempt at humor.

"No, no, no," Patricia shakes her head. "It sounds to me like there has to be a backup system for people. You can do what you do, but they need a backup system and they are not getting it. It's clear to me that when you are with Kate, she's happy that you are there—at least the one time I got to see her."

"She is happy to try while I'm with her, but when I walk away …"

"She does not have the backup system," Patricia finishes. "Because not everybody—I would say probably 60% of the people in this world do not have the same kind of drive that you do. Do you see what I am saying?"

"Yeah."

"So, you want to put your drive into them, but they do not have it. Or, they may have it, but not to the degree that they need it to actually recover from their stroke. You know, stroke advocates can only do so much. Especially if they have been through stroke themselves, they are going to be emotional—they are going to feel the way you do. That's inevitable. So, it is not a failing on your part," Patricia emphasizes.

"Bill, one of the things Sarah and I want to write about is this: how do we educate families and friends to be the kind of support system that the stroke survivor needs them to be? Because I can't be mad at a support person for not having your kind of drive, but I can be mad at the support systems that aren't there." Patricia leans across the table toward Bill, embodying the frustration she has felt as a health communication scholar studying the ways in which missing—or misguided—support leaves patients struggling to live in the aftermath of a health crisis. "Kate's boyfriend isn't doing the exercises with her, the care workers at the house she lives in aren't doing it. It's sad that she doesn't have what you do—that drive—but it's not her failing. It's a failing of a system of friends and family members and health care providers that don't offer the support of following through."

"It's my failing, too, because I should have called the boyfriend," Bill replies, hanging stubbornly on to his sense of culpability. "But I felt like she needed to tell her boyfriend to call me—just call me."

"Yes," Patricia acknowledges, "But guess what? When you're disabled and you don't have the drive, you feel like you're already the biggest burden on this planet—especially because people internalize so much stigma and ableism. So, asking Kate to make that call is like asking Kate to just go ahead and run up the hill right now," Patricia says, gesturing toward the steep road winding up the canyon just beyond her dining room window. "Just go run up that hill!"

"At the same time, family members have to push the stroke survivor to do things for themselves," Bill adds. "Many times, they expect everyone to do everything for them. I get mad and I think, *Get up off your ass and do it yourself.* They'll say, 'Would you hand me that spoon?' and I think, *Well, you can reach over and grab the spoon.*"

"I was watching a couple—the wife cutting up the steak for her husband. Then, she was cutting his desert. I finally stopped them. I said, 'He can do that, let him do that.' And I asked the husband, 'Why are you letting her?' He said, 'Well, I don't want to argue with her.' I said, 'Argue with her! You cut your desert.'"

"It's very difficult," Bill adds, the strident tone of frustration fading away to resignation. "The sad part about me is, I demand of other people to do the same as me—to be reliable, to be persistent. They don't do that, and it sets me up for disappointment. That's a weakness I have, I guess. I set myself up for being disappointed. That hurts me. What can I say?"

THE MUTUAL VULNERABILITY OF BILL'S ADVOCACY WORK

This conversation with Bill reflects the emotional toll that stroke advocacy can take. As a person who has always been guided by a personal code that includes not wasting others' time, being reliable, and being relentlessly persistent, Bill has trouble processing the fact that others do not necessarily operate in this way. Several times over the course of our work together, Bill talked about how the latest disappointment of seeing a stroke survivor stall or regress in their recovery efforts made him question whether or not he should continue with his work. He told us stories of patients who avoided making eye contact with him in hospitals, embarrassed that they had not followed through on his advice. He described making a house call to check on one woman. She pretended not to be home, refusing to answer his repeated knocks at the door.

In interviewing people connected to Bill's story of stroke recovery and advocacy, we had several discussions about the ways in which Bill's approach might not always work—and how these unsuccessful cases affected Bill. In this section, we share snippets of our conversations with Professor Mark Tucker and Charlie Brumfield to explore the limitations of Bill's brand of advocacy.

"THERE ARE OTHER DYNAMICS GOING ON"

"Let me ask you this," Patricia says, sitting in Mark Tucker's office in the Education and Business Administration building at San Diego State. "You have so much expertise in disability and you know a lot about stroke. What is it about Bill you think that allowed him to have a pretty full recovery when a lot of people don't. What do you think it is about him?"

"I think the most salient thing—and a lot of this is coming from my conversations with him—is drive. He's pretty unrelenting in terms of his expectations for himself and maybe, to some extent, his expectations for other folks too."

"And for the book," Patricia jokes, thinking about the persistence with which Bill has brought up the project over the years.

"Yeah," Mark laughs. "He went to the gym every day for a thousand days and I think he attributes a lot of his recovery to that. It certainly is possible that that's a pretty significant factor. Then, in my conversation with him I can see that he sometimes will get sort of frustrated with folks," Mark adds. "He's a believer in that as a strategy that will work for everybody. I think it's a strategy that would have a positive impact for everybody, but I'm not sure it would work as well for everybody else as well as it works for him. To have the drive to go to the gym for a thousand days in a row—If I exercise like 5 days in a row, I feel like that's a pretty big accomplishment for me."

"I know, I know," Patricia laughs.

"So, a thousand days—that's like three years without taking a break. I think that (a), the physical aspect of actually engaging in that was probably a pretty significant contributor to his recovery and then (b), the mindset that's behind that—just his attitude, his orientation. If he's doing that every day, he's also doing all the other stuff that he talks about, like rolling up a towel and rubbing it up and down his face. I've never heard that, and I think that might be a little bit of sort of a folk thing, but he believes it and maybe there is something to that."

"He also was doing okay in life before his stroke. He was a motivated individual, he was a driven individual. Your pre-disability personality and orientation are good predictors of how you're going to do. He was highly motivated, involved, a kind of a go-getter beforehand, so that he would remain that afterward makes a lot of sense."

"One of the dilemma's we're running into …" Patricia begins, picking up on something Mark had hinted at, "and we're not quite sure how to approach it in the book because the book is important to Bill and there's no way that we want to hurt him in any way, but … there's a part of his personality that can make his approach to advocacy very unidimensional." Patricia pauses, choosing her words carefully. "There's a part of me that hopes we can write this in a way to raise his awareness—not just write it, but talk with him about it. We haven't decided how to do it just yet."

"He's probably told you about the woman, Kate he's been working with," she continues. "He's so frustrated. He said, 'I'm not going to meet with her anymore because I come and she's in the same place; she's not working.' I try, little-by-little, to say to him, 'Kate doesn't have support. Her caretaker, her boyfriend, a daughter—nobody's working with her, only you.

You're coming in each week and expecting her to make progress because that's what you did. He accepted that."

Mark nods, understanding Patricia's concerns. "I think of him as a bit like a fitness instructor. He's not a drill sergeant, but the primary flavor that you're getting is that you are the mover and shaker behind your own recovery and you need to pull yourself up by your bootstraps. For him, it has worked exceptionally well. He believes in the power of that approach and, for some folks, it's remarkable. But, you're correct in that for other folks, there are other dynamics going on; they have a different kind of orientation."

"I'm going to relate this a little bit to counseling," Mark says, settling in to professor-style explanation mode. "For somebody like Bill, he's got a lot of self-direction and an internal locus of control[4]—he believes he controls his destiny. I think it's really the predominant approach in our culture; the belief—the narrative—that gets told to everybody, and that we all sort of buy into, to some extent, is that if you succeed it's because of *your* hard work and *your* effort. If you fail, it's also on you."

Patricia laughs, recognizing this sort of narrative in the way that she often thinks about her own successes and shortcomings.

"In some cases that might actually be true," Mark adds. "That tends to be the default way that we approach counseling; we work along with somebody and we hope that a good alliance emerges between the individual and counselor and the two of them, they can accomplish miracles. In some cases, that works. But, if that's the only approach that a counselor adopts, then they're going to run into significant hurdles in working with a large percentage of the population."

---

4. An "internal" locus of control—that is, the belief that much of what happens in life stems from one's own actions—and "external" locus of control—that is, the belief that events in one's life are outcomes of external factors (e.g., fate, luck, other people) and are therefore beyond one's control" (Buddelmeyer & Powdthavee, 2016, p. 89).

"One good example of this is individualistic cultures versus collectivistic cultures.[5] If you are part of a collectivistic culture, the folks who make decisions about your life are not just you. Maybe your parents really are the folks who dictate what happens, or it's an even a broader group of folks that decide what's going on. I can work with you all I want, but we are not going to make any progress until we engage other folks."

"Everybody's involved," Patricia nods, following. "The whole system."

"Right, right," Mark confirms. "I think for folks that have that kind of orientation, it's going to be harder for them to adapt to what Bill's asking them to do. Whereas, for folks who are more from the individualistic orientation, they're going to eat that up. It's going to work really well for them. I see that as probably one of the factors that might explain why somebody with his level of commitment might run into issues with somebody like Kate."

"I don't know Kate, so I don't know exactly what's going on," Mark hedges, "But it wouldn't surprise me if she's maybe a representative of a culture that's more collectivistic; in her life, decisions involve more than just herself. She just feels that everything is under others' control right now. So, then Bill comes in and says, 'no, this is within *your* control.' That will resonate with some people, but others, they're still going to feel significantly *out* of control."

"I think Bill has some appreciation for the importance of relationship dynamics," Mark -adds, shifting topics slightly. "That may be an area where he wanted to magnify his impact. How can I harness the power of the people around this person to facilitate motivation, anticipation, and engagement?"

"Yes, that's good," Patricia says, jotting down notes. "Draw on those other people as resources—pull them in."

"After that, I might start scratching my head and asking, 'Is this person sufficiently depressed that maybe they need professional mental health help?'"

"Through the course of finishing this book," Patricia says, "We want to be able to discuss these dynamics that you're talking about so that people who read the book—and Bill—recognize that there's a wide range of strategies that need to be considered. Because the person's personality before the stroke, or their fitness levels ahead of time, or their individualistic versus the collectivist orientation, or having a network of support or not—all those factors come into play and translate into the way your advocacy strategy must be adapted."

---

5. According to Hofstede, "On the individualist side we find cultures in which the ties between individuals are loose: everyone is expected to look after him/herself and his/her immediate family. On the collectivist side, we find cultures in which people from birth onwards are integrated into strong, cohesive in-groups, often extended families (with uncles, aunts and grandparents) that continue protecting them in exchange for unquestioning loyalty, and oppose other in-groups" (Hofstede, 2011, p. 11).

"YOU GOTTA GIVE WITH NO STRINGS ATTACHED"

"The latest thing we disagree on is interesting," Charlie begins, settling back into the leather couch outside the rehab therapists' offices at Grossmont. "I believe there's a blast site that occurs when a condition arrives in a family setting. Very similar to the Al-Anon[6] and the alcoholic. It goes through all of community. It starts with the children and the significant others and everything, but every single one needs to be communicated with. And even Bill—And I'm gonna tell you something in confidence even though it's on the tape," Charlie adds with his characteristic playfulness. "Bill has a difficult time when he offers his service for free and they won't call back."

"Oh, I know," Patricia agrees. "Yes."

"I gave him my lecture. I go 'Hey, Bill, you gotta give with no strings attached if you want the spiritual benefit of doing it. And what you're facing is, you have an expectation—like expecting your students to go thank you for teaching them how to add. That ain't happening."

"Not frequently anyway," Sarah snorts, remembering the sometimes-thankless work of being a professor.

"So, if you can't get yourself at the spiritual level where you can love without an expectation, there's gonna be a problem. He's so close to being a true spiritual person to begin with," Charlie adds. "He's got a big head start, but it's a bitch when you don't get any feedback. It's so easy for him to persist in his own recovery, but it ain't easy for everybody. And so, if he doesn't get a callback, there's a frustration level. And he's been fighting through that."

"Let me tell you what I see Bill getting that is important to making sure that he can do his work," Charlie says, shifting to discuss the tools Bill draws on to fight through his compassion fatigue.[7] "Number one, he has friends that help him, financially, so he can go do his advocacy work. He's got a car and people donate gas money and things. And that's very important."

"The other thing that I think is important is that his friends have given him some kudos. You're doing it now," Charlie adds, gesturing to Patricia's cellphone voice recorder. "What you're doing is really important to him because no human being is at a point where they can do things without feeling that they're appreciated. So, he's got a nice brochure featuring him at Sharp. He's got a nice book that's gonna feature him. These are things that make the unpaid support possible in the area of stroke survivorship. You have to find a way to do it, and it's hard because there's only so many people who can get a brochure at Sharp Hospital. So, thought needs to go into it. That's the kind of thing that you have to figure out. It's like asking, 'how can you get the person to be recognized for

---

6. Alcoholics Anonymous

7. *Compassion fatigue* (CF) is a term that is used to describe stress that results from "exposure to a traumatized individual rather than from exposure to the trauma itself" (p. 618). CF is often experienced by professionals who are exposed to the trauma of people they serve, such as health care workers, emergency and community service workers, and even family caregivers. Combined with the physical and mental exhaustion in their everyday environment, CF can negatively impact the quality of care provided (Cocker & Joss, 2016).

taking the time to be the referee for the paddleball match without being paid? 'cause all they do is get spit on.'"

"It's like Helen Keller.[8] When you're dealing with the people, you're the Anne Sullivan. How many people will go 'hey, let me sign up for that?' But if you can live through the challenges of doing the advocacy work—even if you don't have success stories like Helen Keller—it teaches you a new way of relating to fellow human beings. It oozes into your entire life."

***

Patricia's phone lights up a moment before her ringer sounds—the pleasingly sweet tones of stroked harp strings. "Hello, Bill," Patricia answers, putting the phone on speaker so Sarah can hear.

"Hi Patricia!" Bill sounds cheerful, energized. "I've got some good news to share!" he says, launching straight into his story. "I was up in a restaurant in Gillespie Field and this man and his wife walked in. I held the door open for them. I saw he had a cane, and I saw his hand was curled up. So, I held a chair for him too and I introduced myself: "My name is Bill. I'm a stroke survivor. I see you had a stroke. I try to do advocacy work and I could come over and maybe I could give you a few exercises that your therapist isn't giving you. You're going to a therapist?'

He says, 'Yes, I go twice a week.'

I say, 'Well, let me give you my card. Here's my website. Call me.' His name was Peter and his wife's name was Mary. I say, 'Now Peter, go ahead and have lunch, thank you. I hope I hear from you.' I know most of the time they never call," Bill adds, a hint of frustration returning to his voice.

"That was two weeks ago. This afternoon, I get a call: 'Bill? This is Peter.'

I say, 'Oh, Peter. How are you?'

He says, 'You remember me?'

I say, 'Sure, you're from Crest. I met you at Gillespie Field.'

He says, 'Great. I've been thinking about what you said and maybe I'll take you up on that offer.'

I said, 'That is wonderful. When can you be available? I'm available any time.'

---

8. Helen Adams Keller was born June 27, 1880, in Tuscumbia, Alabama. After an illness as a young child, Keller became blind and deaf. At the age of 7, her teacher, Anne Sullivan, came to live with Keller's family to help Keller communicate. Keller graduated from college at age 24 and eventually devoted her life to social and political issues, including women's suffrage, birth control, pacifism, and the welfare of blind people. At the age of 40, Keller helped to establish the <u>American Civil Liberties Union</u>. https://www.biography.com/activist/helen-keller

I'm going up to see him Thursday—I'm excited. Sometimes, I get really frustrated. But, I've realized—if I can just help one person, it's worth it."

CLOSING REFLECTIONS

In this chapter, we have explored instances in which Bill becomes frustrated with fellow stroke survivors who either do not follow through on his advice or refuse it entirely. Through our conversations with Professor Mark Tucker, with Charlie, and with Bill, we consider some of the complex dynamics that make Bill's work as a mentor and advocate less straightforward than he might like. Whereas Bill's approach to recovery involved sheer willpower and the ability to transform everyday experiences into rehab exercises, few people have the same penchant for consistency and creativity. Indeed, as Mark noted, some individuals may adopt an external locus of control, rather than the internal locus of control that defines Bill's perspective. In such cases, the individual might believe that the extent of their recovery will be decided by luck, fate, faith, and/or medical skill and technology—not by their own efforts.

Additionally, Bill's recovery story reinforces the assumption that a stroke survivor *can* regain nearly all of their physical and cognitive abilities post-stroke. However, this may not be a possibility for some. Indeed, assuming that all people can and should make a "miraculous" recovery participates in an ableist narrative, reinforcing survivors' feelings of shame and guilt in instances when their symptoms persist.

Additionally, this chapter pushes us to think about how the individualism embedded in Bill's approach to recovery may be ineffective in cases where individuals participate in a more collectivistic family culture or ethnicity. Rather than focusing solely on changing individual behaviors, a more effective strategy might shift the focus to the larger social system of friends and family members in which the person is embedded. How might the important people in a stroke survivor's social circle actually prevent them from making progress in their recovery? How might peer mentors like Bill, and health care providers like recreational therapists and others, transform friends and family members into allies who support the survivor's recovery process? Indeed, advocates like Bill might expand their focus even further, moving beyond working with individuals and their friends and family members to advocating for systemic change in access to acute rehabilitation and other resources.

Finally, this chapter provides an account of Bill's ongoing struggles with compassion fatigue. How does a person like Bill continue to engage in this emotional, time-consuming work in the face of repeated disappointment? Charlie offers us several answers to this question. He urges Bill to resist the desire to place expectations on the people he works with. Instead, he advises Bill to act in good faith, without anticipating any particular outcome. With this advice, Charlie attempts to inoculate his friend against disappointment by focusing his attention on the process, rather than on the result, of helping another person. Additionally, Charlie notes that receiving positive recognition from friends and others helps Bill to remain optimistic. In Chapter 15, we will explore how one hospital system's program for recognizing survivor-advocates plays an important role in validating volunteers like Bill.

REFERENCES

Buddelmeyer, H., & Powdthavee, N. (2016). Can having internal locus of control insure against negative shocks? Psychological evidence from panel data. *Journal of Economic Behavior and Organization, 122*, 88–109. Retrieved from https://www.ncbi.nlm.nih.gov/pmc/articles/PMC5510663/

Cocker, F., & Joss, N. (2016). Compassion fatigue among healthcare, emergency and community workers: A systematic review. *International Journal of Environmental Research and Public Health, 13*, 618–636. https://www.ncbi.nlm.nih.gov/pmc/articles/PMC4924075/

Hofstede, G. (2011). Dimensionalizing cultures: The Hofstede model in context. *Online Readings in Psychology and Culture, 2*, 1–26. https://doi.org/10.9707/2307-0919.1014

CHAPTER 15

"What is *this*?" Sarah asks, flummoxed. She extracts a colorful, glossy magazine from one of the many yellow folders scattered about the living room, holding it up for Patricia to see. A young, glamorously attractive Asian couple poses on the cover, looking superimposed on a background of peach-colored Italian villas on the banks of a Venetian canal. The headlines are written in an unfamiliar, curling script—Thai characters.

Sarah opens the magazine to page 134, squinting at the indecipherable text as if she might suddenly be able to read it. Familiar images are embedded throughout the article—Bill in his red pullover, carrying bags of birdseed toward the lakeshore while ducks and geese follow closely on his heels; Bill holding several pigeons, feeding them with seed from the palm of his hand; a tranquil-looking photograph of Lake Murray. A baby blue thought bubble extends from one picture of Bill, containing the only words printed in English: "When the moon hits your eye like a big pizza pie, that's amore. When the world seems to shine like you've had too much wine, that's amore." Sarah snorts softly, amused by finding the familiar lyrics to one of Bill's favorite songs plopped into the middle of this otherwise indecipherable text.

"Oh!" Patricia says, "Bill told me about the backstory behind this piece. In fact, I think he wrote this one down." She opens another yellow folder, rifling through its contents. "Ah, here it is," she says, triumphantly brandishing one of the blue Calibri accounts that has Bill typed up for us. "This one is called 'Thai Lady at the Lake.'"

THAI LADY AT THE LAKE

One morning while feeding the ducks, I noticed a lady photographing the birds. She walked over to me and asked if she could take pictures of me feeding the birds. I replied, "OK." She took a few pictures and began a conversation. She and her husband were from Thailand and were here on business. She was an amateur photographer and her favorite subject was birds. She asked me about a rare

Contributed by Bill Torres. Copyright © Kendall Hunt Publishing Company.

bird that was seen here at the lake. I said yes, I'd seen it, and if she wanted to take pictures of it, she could come by my car the next morning at 7 a.m. I knew which bird she was talking about because it, along with Gus the Goose and about 50 ducks, would all be waiting for me where I parked my car. The bird—can't remember its proper name—had been visiting the lake for a few days. As usual, he'd heard through the "bird vine" that I was easy pickings. I also learned that he liked to eat in the shade. So, when I moved, the bird would stay in my shadow.

The next morning, after carefully moving 50 or so birds out of the way, I pulled into my usual parking spot. The Thai Lady was watching with amusement. As I was getting out of the car and opening the trunk to get out the food, I noticed the bird in question. I motioned to her to come over next to me and to get her camera ready. She waded through the assorted ducks. I introduced her to Gus the Goose, and I pointed to the bird. I had to calm Gus down because he didn't like people next to me. I had her pet Gus to show she was a friend, and Gus accepted her (suspiciously).

She proceeded to take pictures of the bird. It was intermingled with all the other birds. I asked her if she would like to take pictures of just the bird. Yes was her reply. I moved, and of course my shadow moved with me. The bird followed my shadow (I'd tried this beforehand) and she was amazed! She took about 20 pictures. She asked me how I got the bird to move like that. I eventually told her, and we had a good laugh.

The Thai Lady and I walked down to the edge of the lake, along with Gus and a flock of mallards. She was thrilled to feed the ducks, the geese, and a few squirrels. She asked how I started feeding the ducks. I told it was part of my self- imposed therapy, helping me to recover from a stroke. I was walking at the lake when I noticed a couple of mallards dying from starvation. Their bills had been injured and they had a terrible time trying to eat. I started to hand feed them and, eventually, I started to feed a few more, then a few more, and—finally—all! She was very interested about my stroke. I gave her a condensed version of what happened to me. She asked If I would be at the lake tomorrow. I replied yes. She thanked me and left.

The next day, she came back with her husband. He asked me about my stroke and I gave him the entire story. He asked me for permission to write my story, and I said yes. We continued talking, with him asking me questions. He told me he was a freelance writer. We said our goodbyes, as they were going back to Thailand the next day.

Flash ahead six months. I was feeding the ducks when a young lady asked if I was Mr. Torres. Since she didn't appear threatening, I said yes. She handed me a bag with a magazine inside. She said it was from the Thai couple. Also, it was one of the most popular magazines in Thailand. I said, "Thank you and thank the Thai Couple for remembering me." She took a picture of me holding the magazine. I looked at the magazine. It was very impressive. I opened the magazine to my article. WOW!

A beautiful four-page article with pictures. I later had it translated and it was a beautifully written. It really blew me away. But, wait! Flash forward a few months and the young lady that brought me the magazine surprised me with another edition. This edition contained my picture in the editorial section. Another WOW! I showed Gus the Goose and a few mallards; they weren't impressed!

***

Accounts like 'Thai Lady at the Lake' underline the ways in which telling their story of stroke enables survivors to continue their recovery work and, potentially, their advocacy work. As Charlie noted in the previous chapter, Bill is able to persist in the sometimes-challenging work of mentoring fellow stroke survivors because he continually receives "kudos" from friends and others. In this chapter, we explore how the health care organizations that Bill works with have developed programs that are designed to acknowledge and validate the work of volunteers like him. We focus here on describing Bill's experience as a recipient of Sharp Hospital's Eagle Spirit Award for its 2008 Victories of Spirit dinner. As part of this award, Bill worked with videographer-turned-friend, Randy Stubbs, to recreate his own stroke experience as part of a short video segment that would be screened at the awards banquet. Below, we interview Randy and his colleague, Dan Hanzlik, about the purpose of a program like Victories of Spirit, as well as the process of crafting an awardee's narrative in video form.

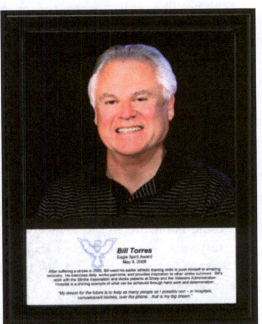

From Sharp HealthCare. Reprinted by permission.

Bill's portrait for the Eagle Spirit Award

VICTORIES OF SPIRIT: ONE HOSPITAL'S PROGRAM FOR RECOGNIZING RESILIENCE

Victories of Spirit is an annual awards banquet hosted by Sharp Memorial Hospital, designed to showcase former rehab patients who have both made significant strides in their own recovery and have also actively given back to the community. Creating this event is a monumental task. A slate of five awardees are selected in October. By January, a team of videographers meets daily, filming interviews with awardees, providers who cared for them, and their friends and family members, recreating scenes from their lives, and editing the footage into short film segments meant to provide a powerfully emotional account of each individual's personal journey.

In our interview with Dan Hanzlik, Manager of Business Development for Sharp Rehab, he described the multiple organizational goals that Victories of Spirit satisfies for Sharp:

> Number one, [Victories of Spirit] is good for the disabled community because it recognizes that there's a large group of people who are disabled who make a decision to give back to that community. That's part of this outreach that we do, just shining that light on the disabled community and what they can do versus what they can't do.
>
> And at the same time, we use Victories of Spirit as a vehicle to shine a light on rehab. Because, in healthcare, rehab is not a sexy diagnosis. It's not a sexy part of healthcare. It's limited in the technological advancement. It's hands-on. It's high-touch versus high-tech. It's not like cardiac, where they're inventing all of this implantable technology. So it's important that we keep that focus in our own community, in our own organization. Victories is now 27 years old, and it's done that. It's been a good advocate for rehabilitation in Sharp, and also in San Diego generally.
>
> Five or six years ago, Sharp as an organization started to recognize the value that this event had. They started bringing big donors or prospective donors to the evenings. We don't ask for money at the event, and we don't charge very much—we call it "friendraising." So, now our foundation brings all these people who are prospective donors and that's how we got a million dollars for the Allison DeRose Rehabilitation center. Robert DeRose is a classic example of somebody who gives back. His daughter had a traumatic brain injury when she was young, and he dedicated his life to helping other people who could not afford to get the help that she received. He and Ray Wallenberg started the survivors' rehab foundation. They've raised over five million dollars, helping 300 or 400 people access rehab who didn't have the money. There are stories like this all over the rehab center.

Dan's description of Victories of Spirit highlights the ways in which stories of survivorship and advocacy work act as an emotional appeal[1] to would-be philanthropists, inspiring them to provide financial support to an otherwise "boring" branch of healthcare, without the use of more direct fundraising tactics like pledge drives and silent auctions. The digital narratives Sharp's team creates, allow audience members to identify with specific "characters," to become invested in their successes, and to see their own stories of personal struggle and triumph reflected in the work that rehab therapists, nurses, and others accomplish.

More than this, however, Dan recognizes the value of simply acknowledging survivors' personal achievements. "I think that there is an abundance of Bills out there," he told us, "They don't all have

---

1. Emotional appeals facilitate persuasion by keeping us engrossed in the story (Baezconde-Garbanati et al., 2014; Moran, Murphy, Chatterjee, Frank, & Baezconde-Garbanati, 2017). Communication researchers have theorized about the persuasive nature of hope appeals in health communication contexts (Chadwick, 2015).

Bill's charismatic personality; sometimes they are doing things that we would consider mundane. There's a gentleman from Grossmont who, after he got hurt, dedicated all of his free time to Momma's Kitchen.[2] Nobody shines a light on people like that—people who are unrecognized but do untold good."

While publicly receiving an award at an event like Victories of Spirit clearly validates the work that peer mentors and advocates do, Randy—the Victories of Spirit videographer—noted that the process of watching their own story unfold on the big screen might actually help individuals to recognize the value of their work. "A lot of people who win these awards, they're very humble; they just live their life and it doesn't seem like any big deal," Randy observed. "Like you," he added, pointing to Sarah, "Your friends will go, 'You're a doctor!' You're like, 'Oh, whatever, yes.' It's just the life that you lived; It's no big deal. But if someone told your story of what you did to become a doctor and you saw it, you'd probably be more proud of yourself and the sacrifices you made to become one. I think

a little of that happens to the Victories of Spirit awardees when their life gets revealed to them in a short time. I think it gives them a little boost of energy, especially if it's someone like Bill Torres who gets picked. It might even make him want to give back more because he sees the effect."

Judging from our own observations of Bill and his advocacy work, Randy's comments are spot-on. Receiving his award at the Victories of Spirit banquet was a turning point moment for Bill, one which solidified his iden-

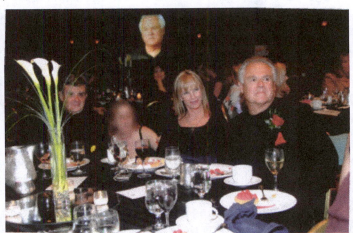

From Sharp HealthCare. Reprinted by permission.

Bill viewing his video with friends at the Victories of Spirit banquet

tity as a stroke advocate. He began to incorporate his Victories of Spirit video in his advocacy work, showcasing it on his website, screening it for students before guest lectures, and sending the link to stroke survivors he intends to work with. For a humble person like Bill, the video became a tool to show others his impressive recovery story without feeling like a braggart. Bill also embraced the dramatic effect he could achieve by showing a video account of his post-stroke paralysis and then striding into a room, appearing completely unencumbered by any lingering stroke symptoms. As a natural showman, Bill recognizes that such a visual contrast—the then-now transformation—serves as a powerful source of hope for stroke survivors still experiencing paralysis, aphasia, and other challenges.

---

2. A San Diego nonprofit whose nutrition services are designed to "improve the lives of women, men, and children vulnerable to hunger due to HIV, cancer, or other critical illnesses." See https://www.mamaskitchen.org/about-us/overview/

Clearly, an event like Victories of Spirit is beneficial, both for advocates like Bill and for health care organizations like Sharp. Yet, as any ethnographer, journalist, or videographer will tell you, telling someone else's story—and getting it right—can be a tricky business. Interviewing someone about their life is an intimate process of getting a person to open up about highly emotional, often painful, experiences. Randy described his process of helping awardees to overcome the nervousness of speaking to a camera surrounded by lights and crew members. "We ask them questions that they know the answers to: How old are you? How many kids do you have? What do you do professionally?" he explained, "Then, we start digging a little deeper into the emotional parts. Once they forget the camera is on, we're just having a conversation. You just try to get the honest truth about their story: What happened? How did they recover? Who helps them recover? What did they learn?" In much the same way that a doctor might attempt to develop a rapport with his or her patient while co-constructing their illness narrative, Randy and his team cultivate interviewees' trust while co-curating their advocacy narrative. Cultivating that level of trust comes with the ethical obligation to tell a survivor's story with care. As Dan told us, the process of publicly sharing such personal narratives may produce some unintended consequences.

"DO NO HARM": MITIGATING THE UNINTENDED CONSEQUENCES OF A SPOTLIGHT

"I am wondering," Patricia begins, sitting across from Dan Hanzlik in his office at Sharp Memorial. "Making these videos, do you see the impact on the folks that you are interviewing?"

"Yes," Dan replies, pursing his lips thoughtfully. "That's an interesting question, actually, because the answer has forced us to re-assess how we do the videos. When we first started doing them— because we were inexperienced—we were trying to make movies. A movie has—you want to grab the person, you want to get their emotions. You want to tell the story, you want the audience to be empathetic, and at the end you want them to feel good and to be uplifted and whatever," Dan explains gesturing with one arm while leaning his elbow on his walnut-colored desk. "We found, at times, that we had to check ourselves to make sure that we did not manipulate the story so that it was either sadder than the person would want to tell it. When we look back, there are few instances where if we had to do it again, we would have done it differently," Dan admits, dropping his head and looking a bit guilty.

"In one case, somebody came forward and said, 'You showed me crying on camera. I would never do that.' They were upset by it. We showed it to 600 people, and the awardee flipped out. Sometimes people are not aware of how raw they are when they are being interviewed. Then when they see it back …," Dan trails off, leaving us to imagine the ways in which screening the results of an intimate conversation might feel like a violation of privacy to an unprepared interviewee. "We had to check ourselves on more than one occasion because this is not Hollywood—this is real life. These are real people who've gone through this. There are so many aspects of the stories that are so fascinating that we have never told. Crazy stuff that you hear and you go, 'Oh, my God. That can't be, but it is.' You couldn't tell that story."

"No," Sarah murmurs, picturing the fallout of outing a person's most explosive secrets via an awards dinner video screening.

"I think we're more—not more honest," Dan pauses, considering his words. "I think we are more careful about that. We try to accomplish the same thing, while realizing that people don't want to be that exposed."

"So that at the end of the day they don't feel used, or they don't feel pushed in a certain direction," Patricia summarizes.

"I think that's exactly right," Dan nods. "We've had arguments about it—the three of us in pro-ducing. It can get volatile—very volatile. We've had times we don't talk to each other at the end of the season," Dan laughs, dispelling the ghosts of old conflicts. "You can't believe how involved you are when you make these things. But I think we are all very careful to try to make sure that we are protecting those folks. I hope when you saw it this year you felt that way," Dan adds, directing this comment at Patricia.

"I did, I did," Patricia reassures him. She pauses for a moment to reflect on attending the *Victories* banquet this year as one of Bill's guests; she remembers the thrill of anticipation that permeated the crowd of elegantly dressed people who mingled before the program began, their high-pitched voices and laughter echoing throughout the decked-out ballroom.

"Do you show these videos to the awardees before the night?" Patricia asks, returning her thoughts to the topic video production.

"No," Dan replies. "Only twice in 65 videos have we ever shown somebody footage ahead of time and it was because it was controversial. I'll give you an example really quick. One of them was about someone who was, in essence, abandoned as a child. They took the community they were involved with now and made them their family. We had this certain point that we put it in the video where we used music, and music is very powerful. So, she says this thing and—boom! we just hit her with this music and it was shocking. It was very dramatic. We made the decision that we were going to have to show that to her and she said, 'No, I don't want that. Even though my parents were terrible to me, I still love them and I don't want to portray them that way.'"

"So, I think I am confident that—even if at the time they might have been embarrassed by some of the emotion, even with the earlier mistakes that we might have made—I think people feel good about it," Dan summarizes, "But it's a big light to shine on somebody." Patricia takes a breath to ask another question, then holds it; there is clearly something else on Dan's mind. "The last thing I am going to say about that is," he begins again. "I often think *Victories* leaves awardees with a void afterward. Because, these are not famous people. They're just folks who are going through their lives and are overcoming big things, but they are not famous and we shine a big light on them.

"And then … nothing," Sarah says.

"Nothing," Dan agrees. "We've worried about that. More increasingly, we've worried about that."

"Is there anything you can do?" Patricia asks.

"That's a good question. Bill did it by becoming more involved."

"He shows the video everywhere!" Sarah laughs.

"Bill's not shy," Dan agrees, smiling. "Bill is that kind of guy that you almost have to put the reigns on him. So, he kind of managed 'the void' that way. But I think, with a lot of people, the bottom drops off when they leave."

"That's a really good point to think about," Patricia says, "I wonder if there might be a plan that would allow someone to maintain a sense of connectedness and not feel that void. I know some of the people show the video in their backyard with a group of friends. It's like a follow-up to the big night."

"That's a good point."

"Or you just prepare them for this," Patricia continues. "They might not realize that they are going to feel that way, kind of like reverse culture shock[3]."

"That's funny, because we talk to them and try to prepare them for it," Dan replies. "We actually meet them the week before with all of our leadership over at corporate. They meet our president, our V.P, and all of the bigwigs and we explain to them, 'Look, you are going to have this attention shined on you. Enjoy it as much as you can.'"

"One of the things that we changed—before I took over in 2008, they would show a much shorter video, about a three-minutes. Then at the end, they would have the person stand up and they would give him a microphone."

---

3. While reverse culture shock typically refers to the emotional and psychological distress suffered by some people when they return to their home culture after living in another culture, a similar form of distress can happen to *Victories* awardees when they return to their "normal" routines after months of being interviewed and filmed for this big event and feel this void created by its absence.

"Oh my gosh," Patricia says in horror, conjuring images of her own terrified public speaking students. "No!"

"It has a lot of potential problems," Dan laughs. "First off, people are either petrified or you can't shut them up. Both are terrible. Second, what I noticed when I went up and talked to the recipients, they weren't even there." Dan passes one hand back-and-forth in front of his unblinking eyes. "They were freaked out. When we got feedback from recipients, one person said, 'I was petrified at speaking and I don't even remember the night. I have no recollection of what happened.'"

"So, we started making the stories longer so they didn't have to tell their story anymore. We tell them, 'Now it's your night. It's your events. You revel in it. You enjoy it. Don't worry about a damn thing, because we are going to tell the story for you.'"

**

This snippet of our interview with Dan reveals important consideration that health care organizations like Sharp must take into account when creating an event to celebrate survivor-advocates like Bill. Does a program that purports to celebrate survivor-advocates simply use individuals' stories for its own fundraising purposes? Without attending to awardee's experience of an event like Victories of Spirit, organizers might unintentionally create embarrassing, even frightening, situations for those they wish to honor. How might an organization's communication professionals balance the need to create emotionally persuasive materials against the ethical mandate to respect an awardee's privacy and preferences? Dan's comments illustrate how he and his team continually review their own processes, seeking input from participants to identify and address the unexpected consequences of their programming (e. g., the post-event "void").

It is clear that, in their approach to "friendraising," the Sharp team foregrounds the needs of survivor-advocates over organizational goals like fundraising. In fact, as Dan explained, the process of getting to know awardees through curating their stories made it impossible not to feel personally invested in getting it "right" for each advocate-survivor. For instance, Dan described how being part of Victories of Spirit shifted the way he views his work. "It really added a level of involvement in the patients in this organization," he explained, "Because I had always been part of the marketing of business aspect of it. I never really connected with them. I was never in the caregiver side, I had nothing to do with it. I was intimidated by disabled people and kind of frightened by them. I didn't know how to talk to them, I didn't know how to respond to people. What really changed that was doing Victories of Spirit." His comments highlight the transformative power of health narratives to connect and to humanize. In our final section of this chapter, we share sections of our interview with videographer, Randy Stubbs, to consider how listening to narratives like Bill's can (re)-shape a person's perspective in powerfully positive ways.

CURATING STORIES, LEARNING LESSONS

"Hello? Randy?" Patricia calls, knocking more firmly on the front door after waiting several minutes for an answer.

"Are we at the right house?" Sarah whispers, looking around skeptically. We've walked up the hill to the end of a what looks like a private cul-de-sac perched on the side of a canyon, following Google's directions to the address that Randy Stubbs had e-mailed to us two weeks earlier. The houses here look more like Airbnb vacation rentals than private homes; there are sundecks with colorfully painted balustrades and tropical decorations. This is our very first interview for the book project with Bill, and this uncertain wait on a stranger's doorstep seems like an inauspicious beginning.

A middle-aged man wearing a ballcap, T-shirt, and running shorts finally appears at the door, squinting through the glass at us. "Hi, it's Patricia Geist-Martin and Sarah Parsloe," Patricia introduces us. "We're here to interview you about Bill Torres."

The man's face transforms. "Oh! I'm so sorry!" Randy exclaims, "I'd forgotten you were coming, and I thought you were some lady I've been having a dispute with. Come in!"

Randy ushers us in to his home, recovering quickly from the shock of finding two mystery women on his doorstep at 9:30 in the morning. We join him in a darkly paneled sitting room outfitted with chocolate leather couches. Tropical decorations adorn this room, too, as well as a series of large movie posters.

"Well I guess we should start by introducing ourselves," Patricia begins after settling on a couch and making sure that the voice recorder on her phone is working. "I teach at San Diego State, and Sarah was my advisee before she went on to get her PhD."

"I went to San Diego State, too." Randy says. "I used to be a Special Education teacher—that's actually what I graduated in. I had a roommate at that time down in Mission Beach. He was a surfer and he wanted me to take pictures of him surfing. He showed me the basics. I went out there, shot him surfing, and went to San Diego State to the photo lab. These pictures started magically coming up. Capturing that one moment that will never happen again and being able to preserve it, enhance it, and save it—I was just lost in the magic of that, and I went back and got a degree in photo journalism. Photo journalism is telling a story; it's exactly what you're doing here with your book project, except that, as a photojournalist, you're doing it visually."

"Yes," Patricia agrees, "the editing process is going to be similar, too—figuring out what we take out of these stories and what we keep."

"Exactly," Randy nods. "It's the same thing with different media. It was funny that I started doing stuff like Sharp and United Way-ish, non-profit stuff because I always liked the emotional connection. It's all about the emotional. I started working for Mercy Hospital. They have a program like Victories of Spirit called Miracles of Mercy. Then, I came over to Sharp—I think this is my 17th year."

"Wow!"

"I have about four other consistent jobs that are little less heavy duty," Randy adds. "Like we're doing a skit right now for this company, like a 1960s Batman."

"That's a little different than Victories of Spirit!" Patricia laughs.

"Yes, it's a nice break to perk me back up. It's pretty heavy duty with all those stories"

"Just a side note. My niece doing stunts in a new *Pirates of the Caribbean* light show that's going to open this month at Disneyland," Patricia says, pointing to a framed *Pirates* movie advertisement on the wall behind her.

"I love *Pirates of the Caribbean*!" Randy says, nerding out. "In fact, that pirate thing up there, it was from that restaurant, Blue Bayou. They were remodeling it and I happened to be there the last day that they would be open for the next year. They gave the menus away. That was actually the other side of the menu."

"That's awesome!" Sarah enthuses.

"Yep. Anyway, anything else you want to know about me?"

"Could you tell us the story of when you first met Bill?" Sarah asks. "How did you meet? What was your first impression of him?"

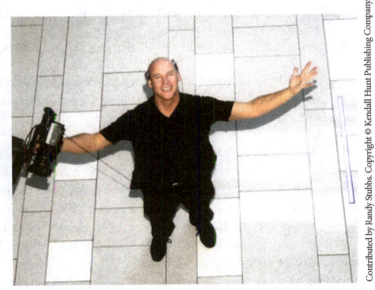

Randy Stubbs, Sharp videographer

"He was a recipient of Victories of Spirit. I remember those interviews—we actually shot them at Sharp in an office building or something. I remember looking down the hallway and seeing this guy talking to my Sharp people. They were prepping him for filming. He was nothing like I thought when I read the description of his story. I thought he was going to be this feeble guy. He really didn't have too many signs of having a stroke or anything."

"He was a really good interviewee because he just let the truth out. That's the thing—we want the truth. He had no problem doing that. At the time, I hadn't done too many stroke survivor videos. So, I didn't really know a lot about strokes. I learned a lot about strokes through interviewing Bill. I remember immediately just being impressed with what a great interviewee he was and just how dynamic he was."

"Did you watch the video with Bill after you filmed his story? What was his response?"

"I don't think I've ever watched Bill's with him. In fact, when he was at the event, he said he barely paid attention to it when they were playing it because it's nerve-racking. You sit there and there's 500 people in there watching your story. He only watched it in your class, Patricia. It's when he really started to listen to what he said."

"Yes, he said he didn't want to be there when I showed the video to the class," Patricia laughs. "He said, 'I want the drama of me walking in after they've seen it.'"

"You need to add some smoke for his entrance," Randy jokes, poking fun at Bill's theatrical flair.

"That reminds me of a question I wanted to ask you," Patricia segues. "You don't remain close friends with every Victories of Spirit awardee. Why do you think you and Bill have kind of maintained the friendship over the years?"

"We have a lot in common. We think similarly about what's important in life, I think. We're not materialistic," Randy pauses, considering. "We have just this great connection. He's a guy you feel you want to help because he helps so many people and the birds and everything. He does so much without asking for anything. We have a mutual friend, George. He's not really a philanthropist, but he has a lot of money. He likes to help people. He's the one that bought Bill his Fiat. He met Bill and heard Bill's story, and George saw that this guy is worthy of being helped. Look at what he's doing for no money. He's the one that pays for Bill's gas. It allows Bill to help more people because he can afford to drive all over. George doesn't even really understand that. He's 90, but he doesn't really understand how much that helps Bill. Because he has a lot of money, he can't understand."

"Bill had that. Bill had fancy cars and big houses and everything like that. He was in-between insurances I think when the stroke happened. He lost everything. It probably stung for a while, but he doesn't let it affect his life. He adjusted pretty fast—I think he reprioritized what's really important."

"I think these videos from Victories of Spirit, they're so meaningful because they tell life lessons like that," Randy adds, turning contemplative. "Because I think, in life, we learn all those lessons through our family. People die, loved ones have injuries and stuff like that, but it's a slow process over decades. A guy from *Victories* last year, he was 17 years old and broke his neck in a motorcycle race. All those lessons—what's really important in life—it's concentrated in three years. That guy grew up in three years. I think the part of the night at *Victories* that is the most rewarding is all the lessons people get to learn almost vicariously through other peoples' stories. You can't help but put a little part of that in your own life."

"Everything to me is a lesson," Randy continues. His gestures become more animated as he warms up to this subject. "Personally, how these stories have helped me is thinking about death. Everyone has deaths in their family. I lost my grandmother, my mother, my sister, my dad, my aunt, our dog that we grew up with—everything—all in five years. No one had ever died before that. It was like, Boom, boom, boom, boom," Randy karate chops one hand against his open palm, emphasizing the emotional violence that he experienced. "You're overwhelmed at first," he acknowledges. "But then I've come to the conclusion that if there isn't a lesson then their life—there has to be a lesson in their death."

"I'll tell you a great story about my mom," Randy continues, echoing the same enthusiasm Bill often shows for telling a good tale. "My sister died at 49 of cancer. Three years after my sister's death, my mom was doing a crossword puzzle and she just had to stretch out over our thick, green shag carpet. She was sitting there, and she goes, 'I'm done.'

I go, 'Oh, did you finish your crossword puzzle?'

She goes, 'No, I just decided I'm done being sad about Kim. I don't totally believe that she's floating up there looking down and watching everything I do and stuff. But if in some capacity, she could see what I'm doing, I felt like I needed to be sad to reflect how much I cared about her and how deep the loss is. But from this day forward, I choose happiness because I'm going to honor her. If she can see me, she would want me to be happy. So, I'm going to honor her life by choosing happiness."

"Another neat story, a lesson," Randy continues, chaining across the connected narratives of his life. "When my mom died, she donated her body to medical research as all my family did. So, there's no burial, no cremation. I didn't plan it, but I cut off a couple of lumps of her hair. I gave one to my brother and one to me."

"I was crew on a sailboat at the time. In fact, I was crewing for a guy that used to be a Victories of Spirit winner that had his legs amputated and still sails his boat. I just went to the bow of the boat I threw these flowers and mom's hair over. Every time we'd race the same waters, my friend would say, 'Sacred waters.' I'd feel sad because it was like saying goodbye to my mom again."

"One time, six months later, he said, 'Sacred waters. Oh, my God!' We look, and there's 10 or 20 yellow flowers in the water, just like the flowers I threw out from the bow. In this big ocean, we go right through someone else's yellow flowers."

"For the first time, instead of saying goodbye to my mom, I said, 'Hello.' It was like that," Randy gestures as if he is flipping a light switch. "It was this big thing. Then, going through sacred waters was a happy thing. Every time we would go through there, I'd be happy to say, 'Hello, Mom.'"

"It's those little lessons in life that I don't think I would've been receptive to if I hadn't done these videos," Randy concludes, returning to his work as a videographer for Victories of Spirit. "I don't think I would have learned these as deeply. Because I know how these heavy things are going to affect your life and ruin it, if you let them. So, there has to be a lesson there."

CLOSING REFLECTIONS

In this chapter, we have explored how Sharp's Victories of Spirit program offers an important opportunity to tell survivor-advocates' stories and validate their achievements. As Randy noted, the processes of being interviewed, filming recreated scenes from their life, and watching their own story on the big screen can serve as an important sense-making resource of individuals who may not have fully recognized the value of their own narrative. Indeed, as Matthews and Sunderland (2017) note, celebrity and public events like *Victories* create important listening environments. They write that "storytelling in intimate spaces and moments can be the glue that cements a new relationship or reinforces an advocacy network's resolve to continue their work" (p. 18). For a person like Bill, participating in Victories of Spirit affirmed his advocate identity, providing both renewed energy and a communication tool with which to continue his work.

However, as our conversation with Dan revealed, the process of telling people's story on their behalf—particularly in a public setting—is fraught with potential pitfalls. Dan, Randy, and their team members act as "curators," producing and arranging a series of survivor-advocate stories. "Curated collections are often themed or fit within a metanarrative and may be gathered together with a particular purpose in mind" (Matthews & Sunderland, 2017, p. 26). As such, curatorship is a purposeful, active process in which the curator has power to (re)shape a person's story in the process of (re)presenting it. As Dan noted, organizational purposes—such as the desire to tell emotionally persuasive narratives that demonstrate the value of rehab and encourage philanthropic donations—may come in conflict with the desire to protect awardees' privacy and acknowledge the emotional vulnerability inherent in their sharing publicly the personal challenges they have experienced. In addition, the institutionalized listening context of *Victories* mandates an emotional tone of celebration. As a result, the process of curating and editing survivor-advocates stories to evoke inspiration may censor the frustrations that often emerge from issues within the health care system—such as limited access to acute rehabilitation—that would be a more transformative foci for advocacy work (Matthews & Sunderland, 2017).

Finally, our conversation with Randy revealed the very personal impact of listening to, and re-presenting, a survivor-advocates story. He describes the lessons he learned through interviewing, editing, and screening *Victories* videos over many years. These are the same kinds of lessons that Patricia's students respond to whenever Bill gives a guest lecture in her class. In the epilogue for this book, we explore how our work with Bill—listening to his stories and figuring out how to represent his life—deeply affected us.

REFERENCES

Baezconde-Garbanati, L., Chatterjee, J. S., Frank, L. B., Murphy, S., Moran, M. B., Werth, L. N., . . . O'Brien, D. (2014). *Tamale Lesson:* A case study of a narrative health communication intervention. *Journal of Communication in Health Care, 7,* 82–92.

Chadwick, A. E. (2015). Toward a theory of persuasive hope: Effects of cognitive appraisals, hope appeals, and hope in the context of climate change. *Health Communication, 30,* 598–611. doi: 10.1080/10410236.2014.916777

Matthews, N., & Sunderland, N. (2017). *Digital storytelling in health and social policy: Listening to marginalised voices.* New York, NY: Routledge.

Moran, M. B., Murphy, S., Chatterjee, J. S., Frank, L. B., & Baezconde-Garbanati, L. (2017). The power of storytelling to improve health outcomes. In J. Yamasaki, P. Geist-Martin, & B. F. Sharf (Eds.), *Storied health and illness: Communicating personal, cultural, and political complexities* (pp. 283–285). Long Grove, IL: Waveland.

COMMUNICATION LESSONS LEARNED

In *Part Three* of this book, we have explored the ways Bill communicates as an advocate and peer mentor. These chapters are rife with communication lessons, but we focus on five. We begin by discussing essential communication competencies—including listening actively and empathetically, mindful patient-centered care, reciprocity, and modeling. We offer examples of how Bill practices these in his encounters with stroke survivors and their family members. We also draw on some additional theoretical concepts to illuminate reasons why Bill's approach to working with stroke survivors is sometimes ineffective. Finally, we incorporate health narrative scholarship to consider the ways Bill's narrative framing of his own stroke recovery journey informs his advocacy work.

Our first communication lesson focuses on the valuable role that active-empathic listening plays in advocating or offering help to others. Active-empathic listening behaviors are defined as "a set of behaviors that function to demonstrate attention, understanding, responsiveness, and empathy; to encourage continued expression of thoughts and feelings; and to aid in relational maintenance" (Thompson, 2014, p. 1364). These behaviors include listening to both *what* is said and *how* it said, asking questions and paraphrasing to check understanding, and responding without appropriating or invalidating another person's comments. Too often, people do not engage in active-empathic listening. As Stephanie Ousley from Grossmont Hospital noted, unsuccessful peer advocates have the tendency to seek opportunities to tell their own story and express their own perspective, rather than asking questions to better understand the perspective of the person they are seeking to assist. This approach to peer mentorship might be described as a form of "conversational narcissism," defined as "an extreme self-focusing in a conversation," including "refocusing the topic of conversation on the self" (Vangelisti & Knapp, 1990, p. 251). In contrast, Bill makes use of active-empathic listening. For instance, instead of seeking opportunities to refocus the conversation on his own story, Bill uses his vivid memories of recovering from stroke as a tool for empathy—as a device for making sense of and responding to another person's physical and emotional challenges. Additionally, active-empathic listening involves nonverbal immediacy behaviors, such as making eye contact, leaning forward, and touching, that reduce the psychological distance between two communicators (Thompson,

2014). As David Brown told us, "Bill will touch—he's not a distance away. He'll hold your hand, he'll put his hand on your arm … He touches you, which brings a level of comfort."

Our second lesson draws our attention to the importance of being a mindful, patient-centered communicator. The BATHE model (Miller, 2004; Stuart & Lieberman, 2002)., used as a training tool for health care providers, provides a handy acronym of the questions and statement that caregivers (or any support provider) might utilize to accomplish this form of communication:

Background: What is going on in your life?

Affect: How do you feel about that? What is your mood?

Trouble: What troubles you about that?

Handling: How are you handling that?

Empathy: That must be very difficult for you.

We can observe Bill enacting some of the steps of BATHE in many of his advocacy stories, including his account of working with the married couple John and Marsha. Bill carefully asked each spouse questions to elicit their emotional states (**B**ackground and **A**ffect) and understand the source of their distress (**T**rouble). He asked Marsha to walk him through her approach to mealtime (**H**andling) and validated her frustration (**E**mpathy), even though he arrived at their home fairly confident that he already understood the problem.

A third communication lesson is the power of reciprocity (Cialdini, 2009); when someone gives us something, we feel obligated to respond in kind. Stories like the John and Marsha tale illustrate that Bill is most successful when he gains the buy-in of those he is trying to assist. Randy's comments revealed how this basic principle of persuasion functions in Bill's work as an "independent contractor." He explained, "Here's a guy who does not get paid; he's doing this out of the goodness of his heart …. [The stroke survivors he works with think] *Wait, this guy has come and he's caring about me. He's doing more for me than my family members are doing.* I think, maybe, they almost feel a little obligation to try and listen to him". Indeed, Bill capitalizes on the norm of reciprocity in his attempt to inspire stroke survivors to "pay it forward" after they recover. Randy told us that Bill "compels" stroke survivors to give back, telling them, "If you ever get better, you're one of the lucky ones. You should go and help other people. Because no one knows the story like you know the story."

A fourth, related communication lesson in advocacy work highlights the importance of individuals modeling the behaviors that they want the stroke survivor to perform. According to social learning theory, "By observing a model of the desired behavior, an individual forms an idea of how response components must be combined and temporally sequenced to produce new behavioral configurations" (Bandura, 1971, p. 8). Bill models his own strategies for fellow stroke survivors, showing them how simply inserting a key into a lock might become a valuable rehabilitation exercise. As several of our interviewees observed, Bill is effective because he physically represents a model of stroke recovery. Bill frequently instructs health care staff to introduce him before he enters the room, describing the seriousness of his strength and the length of his recovery process. He capitalizes on the element of surprise he can achieve by walking in after such a description. "What he's doing is trying to give them hope," Randy told us. "Because they see him as shining example, walking and joking around."

A fifth important lesson is the critical importance of adapting supportive communication to meet the survivors' needs. In fact, health communication scholars have focused on the importance of framing supportive messaging so they match with people's support needs (Cutrona, 1990; Goldsmith, 2004). Bill's approach to working with stroke survivors is not always effective, often causing him to experience compassion fatigue. For instance, while Bill might provide a person like Kate with emotional support, encouraging her to think positively about her chances of recovery, what she may really need is tangible support (e.g., access to additional therapy).

Finally, a sixth lesson from Part Three of this book reveals the ways health narratives can serve as tools for advocacy and peer mentorship. Frank (1995) describes different types of stories that survivors might tell, including what he terms restitution, chaos, or quest narratives. In working with stroke survivors, people serve as co-narrators, helping individuals to make sense of their own experiences. As a co-narrator, Bill uses his work with the hand acts as a sense-making device; he narrates the process of rehabilitating the brain through a seemingly insignificant task of finger straightening. Bill constructs his own story of recovery using the "restitution narrative" (Frank, 1995); it is a relatively uncomplicated tale of experiencing a health crisis, working diligently to address devastating symptoms, and achieving a triumphant return to his previously able-bodied self (with a few lingering challenges). This restitution narrative is particularly compelling and inspiring to stroke survivors and their families who feel stuck in a "chaos narrative" (Frank, 1995). In their chaos narrative, survivors struggle to make sense of an unpredictable, uncontrollable body that refuses to cooperate with efforts to return to "normal."

However, Bill's reliance on a restitution narrative may be problematic for some, particularly when their experience of recovering from a stroke is untidy and unpredictable, and when complete recovery may not be a possibility. In fact, the real value in telling a story like Bill's may lie in his telling of a "quest narrative" (Frank, 1995). Recounting the struggles and successes Bill experienced over a lifetime, focuses attention not on the fact that he made a "miraculous" recovery, but instead on the valuable lessons he has learned in living a messy life. The man who once drove sports cars and wore Armani suits now drives a Fiat donated by an aging millionaire and often wears a faded red jacket coated with birdseed dust. Yet Bill has gained, as Charlie phrased it, "a new way of relating to fellow human beings" that "oozes into [his] entire life."

REFERENCES

Bandura, A. (1971). *Social learning theory.* New York, NY: General Learning Corporation.

Cialdini, R. B. (2009). *Influence: Science and practice* (5th ed.). Boston, MA: Pearson Education, Inc.

Cutrona, C. E. (1990). Stress and social support—in search of optimal matching. *Journal of Social and Clinical Psychology, 9,* 3–14. doi:10.1521/jscp.1990.9.1.3

Frank, A. (1995). *The wounded storyteller: Body, illness, and ethics.* Chicago, IL: The University of Chicago Press.

Goldsmith, D. J. (2004). *Advances in personal relationships. Communicating social support.* New York, NY: Cambridge University Press.

Miller, W. (2004). The clinical hand: A curricular map for relationship-centered care. *Family Medicine, 3,* 330–335.

Stuart, M. R., & Lieberman, J. A., III. (2002). *The fifteen-minute hour: Practical therapeutic interventions in primary care* (3rd ed.). Philadelphia, PA: Saunders.

Thompson, T. L. (2014). *Encyclopedia of health communication.* Thousand Oaks, CA: Sage.

Vangelisti, A. L., & Knapp, M. L. (1990). Conversational narcissism. *Communication Monographs, 57,* 251–274. doi:10.1080/03637759009376202

EPILOGUE

FALLING IN LOVE WITH THE PROCESS

"Well, last week Philip the Goose quit coming up to the parking lot to see me," Bill reports as he parks in his usual spot at Chollas Lake. "He wasn't waiting at the car. I'd see him down by the lake, so I'd say, 'Philip, what's wrong? Why aren't you meeting me up here?'" He pauses as we climb out of the Fiat, waiting until we meet again by the back bumper. "Well, he has a girlfriend," Bill explains, opening the car's trunk to retrieve bags of birdseed and peanuts. "Yesterday, he brought his girlfriend to meet me. It was so cute! They came up to me and I fed both of them. That made me feel so good, because Philip just had ignored me for a week." Bill is talking about birds, but his words seem to hold greater significance. They hint at the pain of finding oneself abandoned in relationships with others; they capture the joy of rekindling a connection. As Bill turns toward the lake, a pigeon lands on his shoulder. A squirrel emerges from under a tree root and a brown goose waddles up to join them. Bill grabs a handful of seed and extends his palm, unfurling his fingers. As he reenacts this daily ritual of caring for others, he finds himself falling even deeper in love with the process.

***

When we began writing this book, we envisioned writing a classically academic, ethnographic piece, applying concepts from health communication scholarship to understand how individuals cultivate resilience as they move through health crises. In some ways, we have accomplished this. We have provided accounts of how communication processes like developing and maintaining a social network, providing and receiving social support, listening and being listened to, and bolstering one's own and others' sense of self-efficacy can contribute to better health outcomes post-stroke. For stroke survivors and those who love them, we hope that this book offers bits of practical advice. We'd also like readers to recognize that attaining a "miraculous" recovery isn't as important as surrounding themselves with others who support them in setting the small, daily, manageable challenges that keep them focused on achieving what is most functionality possible for their bodies. At the same time, these supporters are critical in moving forward psychologically and emotionally.

While this book has fulfilled some of our expectations, it has also become something more than what we had anticipated. In writing about how stroke survivors might, as Peter Levine (2013) encouraged, "fall in love with the process" of recovery, we fell in love with the process of writing—the process of getting to know Bill and recounting his life stories. Like the Sharp videographer, Randy Stubbs, we learned that the process of curating another person's narrative inevitably re-shapes your own. It leaves you with the sense of having gained important life lessons by having lived vicariously through someone else's story. As we conclude this book, we offer our own accounts of how our interactions with Bill affected us.

KNOWING BILL: PATRICIA'S STORY

I have to admit—when I first met Bill, he seemed a bit creepy. When he approached me and my girlfriends after our lakeside workout, he seemed like an eccentric animal lover who was, perhaps, a bit too friendly for comfort. Yet, as Bill began collaborating with me as a guest lecturer in my class, our relationship blossomed. Every phone call to plan his visit, every class presentation, and every post-lecture breakfast to debrief and plan for future visits was a joyful accumulation of memories with Bill. Bill is over a decade younger than my father would be by now. However, because I lost my father to heart disease when I was 33 and he was 71, my memories of him are frozen at the age he was when he died. Bill was 73 when we met—so close to my father's age. As we got to know one another, I felt this deep fatherly connection. My dad and I were close; closer than most, since he was my touchstone after my mom died of cancer when I was 17. Bill has become a marvelous father figure in my adulthood, filling the huge gap that my father left in my life. I truly care about Bill—I want to know what he's doing, how he's feeling, and when we're going to see each other again.

Throughout the process of writing of this book, I could call Bill on the spur of the moment and he would answer immediately or call back within the hour. While our conversations used to focus solely on getting answers to questions about the book, it's been fun to just talk about anything else happening in our lives. Recently, I found a baby mockingbird that had fallen out of the tree in my backyard. When I called, Bill came right over with a special box for carrying birds and offered to take the little one to Project Wildlife.[1] We sat together in my backyard and watched the little bird for a short while, witnessing its mother drop bits of food in her fuzzy, chirping baby's outstretched mouth. It broke both our hearts to take the bird away from its mother, but we knew it would never survive on the ground with cats and coyotes roaming the neighborhood. So, off Bill went with the bird. He called with an update 30 minutes later, telling me that the wing was broken and that the staff would nurse the baby back to health and release it back to nature.

A turning point moment in our relationship occurred when Bill called me to tell me his idea for a new title for the book. He had already talked with Sarah and discovered that she loved it; now he

---

1. See https://www.sdhumane.org/programs/project-wildlife/

was running it by me. I was thrilled when he offered some great ideas about what to include in the chapter I was working on.

"Bill, you are just so smart, this is perfect!" I blurted. For a moment, there was silence on the other end of the phone line. "Bill, are you okay?" I asked. I could hear that he was struggling with tears.

"Oh, Patricia," Bill said. "That means so much to me that you said that—that you think I am smart. I always think of myself as having practical smarts, but not book smarts like you."

"Oh, Bill, you are so smart. This book is as great as it is because of you and because of all your insight."

We talked for a little while longer. As we said our goodbyes, Bill said through tears, "You know that I love you, Patricia."

"I love you too, Bill—I mean that. I love you."

KNOWING BILL: SARAH'S STORY

An e-mail notification pops up on my phone—a message from Bill with the cryptic subject line, "20180527_065157.jpg." I click to open it:

Bill Torres: Here's a friend I haven't seen in 2 years

Sarah Parsloe: Beautiful! You recognize the markings? What's his/her name?

Bill Torres: I never gave him or her a name. I recognized its markings and she immediately flew to me. Maybe I'll call her Sarah, would you mind?

Sarah Parsloe: I wouldn't mind! I think it's fitting, given that we both leave for long periods, but always fly back.

Bill Torres: It's also fitting that she is young and beautiful. Am I not coo-rect?

Sarah Parsloe: Don't pigeonhole me. Beauty is a bird-un 😊

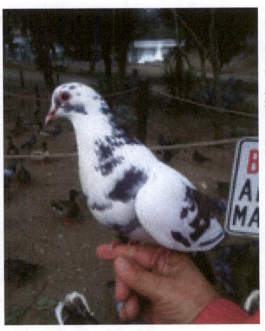

Bill Torres: Didn't mean to ruffle your feathers. I'm just a birdbrain!

I smile as I read Bill's final e-mailed response; this kind of witty verbal jousting is typical of our relationship. To Bill, I likely seem very much like Sarah the Pigeon, disappearing for months at a time and reappearing unexpectedly. Yet, from my perspective, I am always with him in the process of writing. I pour over transcripts of our recorded conversations, re-imagining and, consequently, reliving our visits together. Periodically, Patricia sends recordings of new conversations she's had with Bill in my absence. As I listen to their taped voices, I feel like I am a voyeuristic presence in the room with them, laughing—unseen and unheard—as I listen to Bill recount yet another large-than-life coincidence story. As I render our raw transcripts into polished narratives, I feel as if I have been a similarly voyeuristic witness to Bill's life, living with him through the Great Depression, the San Diego racquetball boom, the terrifying day of his stroke, and the triumphant moment of help-ing Delray take his first few steps unaided by a wheelchair. Just like a stroke survivor who Bill has helped, but who he rarely hears from, I am affected by having known Bill in more ways than he likely realizes. I write as an indirect way of thanking him, knowing that he will read these words sometime in the future, on opposite sides of our shared continent.

***

My phone dings, notifying me of a new message from Patricia. A recording is attached—the one I've been waiting for. I feel a bit nervous as I download the MP4 file on my computer and click the triangular "play" icon.

"When I got home, it was burning a hole in my car seat," Bill's familiar voice says, referring to the printed copy of our draft book manuscript that Patricia had given him to read. "I set it down and I stared at it. I looked at it and I said, 'Well, this is an academic thing.' I attack fiction reading different than I attack nonfiction reading, and I attack textbooks differently. I was confused about how to attack it. So, I said, 'I'm just going to read it and try to enjoy it, but still edit it.'"

"That's hard to do!" I hear Patricia say.

"Yeah! And …" Bill's voice hesitates. "It was wonderful. I tried to still separate myself from it and think, *I'm reading about this character.* And I do have a lot of stories, huh?"

"You do, you do!" I hear Patricia's enthusiastic agreement.

"Anyway, it was just wonderful how both of you just made a beautiful tapestry. And it was just there, glowing. It was … you know I was watching TV, I was watching Jeopardy, and I said, 'I've got to dis-tract myself in some way so that I don't get too emotional and I really can't read it.' So, I was trying to keep the emotions at bay, and it was very difficult—especially when I started reading Russell's story, and I'm going, 'God, I remember seeing him eating that sandwich there in the hospital and feeling sorry for himself.' So then, I started creating other stories!"

I can hear Patricia laugh on the recording. I imagine that she must have been bracing herself to hear yet another story that we'll need to weave into the book.

"'I go, 'Can't do that! Must concentrate!'" Bill's voice continues. "I'd give up and walk around and talk to the skunk outside and talk to the opossum. So, anyway, I just had a wonderful time reading, and I love both of you. What can I say?" Bill's voice wavers. I picture his eyes filling with tears. I hear the telltale tap of a hand patting someone's back as Patricia and Bill embrace.

"I love you, too, Bill," Patricia's voice says.

"It just blows my mind. I still can't believe that the book is about me—it's very difficult, very difficult. And the nice things people said … I don't have words. I have emotions. And when I leave here I'll go home and cry and get it out of my system because … Damnit, Sarah, why aren't you here?" Bill's voice is suddenly louder as he turns toward the recorder.

I'm here, Bill. I hear you.

***

My phone alerts me of yet another new e-mail in my inbox. Bill has titled this one less cryptically: "Sarah has returned."

Bill Torres: Look who returned. She still recognizes me. I let her read one of the chapters. Her response was, "cooooool!"

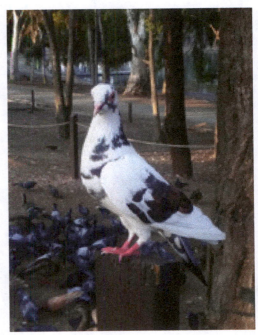

Contributed by Bill Torres. Copyright © Kendall Hunt Publishing Company.

REFERENCE

Levine, P. G. (2013). *Stronger after stroke: Your recovery roadmap to recovery* (2nd ed.). New York, NY: demosHEALTH.

CPSIA information can be obtained
at www.ICGtesting.com
Printed in the USA
FSHW020100241019
63325FS